Clinical Computed Tomography for the Technologist

Second Edition

Clinical Computed Tomography for the Technologist

Second Edition

Lee C. Chiu, M.D.
Clinical Professor
University of California
Los Angeles, California
St. Joseph's Medical Center
Burbank, California

James D. Lipcamon, R.T.(R)
Chief Technologist
Jennie Edmundson Memorial Hospital
Council Bluffs, Iowa

Victoria S. Yiu-Chiu, M.D.
Ultrasound Division
Long Beach Memorial Medical Center
Long Beach, California

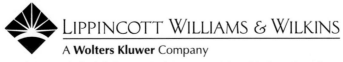

LIPPINCOTT WILLIAMS & WILKINS
A **Wolters Kluwer** Company
Philadelphia • Baltimore • New York • London
Buenos Aires • Hong Kong • Sydney • Tokyo

Printed in the United States of America

Library of Congress Cataloging-in-Publication Data

Clinical computed tomography for the technologist / authors, Lee C. Chiu, James D. Lipcamon, Victoria S. Yiu-Chiu ; with a contribution from Diane O'Dell.—2nd ed.
    p. cm.
  Rev. ed. of: Clinical computed tomography / Lee C. Chiu, James D. Lipcamon, Victoria S. Yiu-Chiu. 1986.
  Includes bibliographical references and index.
  ISBN 0-7817-0235-6
  1. Tomography. I. Chiu, Lee C. II. Lipcamon, James D. III. Yiu-Chiu, Victoria S. IV. O'Dell, Diane. V. Chiu, Lee C. Clinical computed tomography.
  [DNLM: 1. Tomography Scanners, X-Ray Computed. WN 160 C6402 1995]
  RC78.7.T6C45 1995
  616.07′572—dc20
  DNLM/DLC
  for Library of Congress   94-3656

9 8 7 6 5 4

Contents

v

Contributors

Lee C. Chiu, M.D.
Clinical Professor
University of California,
Los Angeles, California
St. Joseph's Medical Center
501 South Buena Vista Street
Burbank, California 91505

Victoria S. Yiu-Chiu, M.D.
Ultrasound Division
Long Beach Memorial Medical Center
2801 Atlantic Avenue
Long Beach, California 90801

James D. Lipcamon, R.T.(R)
Chief Technologist
Jennie Edmundson Memorial Hospital
933 Pierce Street
Council Bluffs, Iowa 51502

Diane O'Dell, B.S.R.T.
Department of Radiology
University of North Carolina at Chapel Hill
School of Medicine
Chapel Hill, North Carolina 27514

Foreword

Since the advent of computed tomography (CT) during the early 1970s, many books have been written about various aspects of the procedures. This book was truly needed, as it is one of the most complete covering CT for technologists.

Lee C. Chiu, James D. Lipcamon, and Victoria S. Yiu-Chiu have successfully integrated the anatomy and technique of computed tomography into chapters representing the various body areas. In addition, they have devoted chapters to such important topics as contrast media used in CT, clinical considerations, and CT-guided biopsies, as well as a basic introduction to CT.

Practicing technologists will find this to be an invaluable book for acquiring the knowledge and skills used to produce diagnostic CT examinations.

Marilyn Holland, B.S., R.T
Director
Radiologic Technology Education
University of Iowa Hospitals and Clinics
Iowa City, Iowa

Preface

Computed tomography (CT) continues to evolve as an important diagnostic tool in the radiological armamentarium. This evolution continues as a result of advancements in hardware and software. Just when it appears that CT has closed its final chapter, a new technological advancement starts a new one, such as the case with spiral CT. As more is expected from CT, technologists in the field will need to be more knowledgable about this modality. In many hospitals and clinics, technologists are expected to make decisions that affect the technical quality of an examination. These decisions frequently are based on knowledge of normal cross-sectional anatomy. This book was developed out of what we found to be a void in resources designed specifically for the technologist with reference especially to cross-sectional anatomy.

In addition to the cited references in the text, we have included suggested readings that the reader will find interesting and informative.

This book provides a thorough introduction to normal cross-sectional anatomy and techniques for the most commonly performed examinations. The cranial and extracranial regions of the body are discussed making this a versatile book for the technologist. The book should serve not only as a teaching instrument but also as a working clinical guide and reference source.

Lee C. Chiu
James D. Lipcamon
Victoria S. Yiu-Chiu

Acknowledgments

Production of this book would not have been possible without the assistance of many people. A special thanks goes to Cathy Hughes who spent hours typing and revising our manuscript. We would like to thank Deeanna and Don Hockett for their excellent work in preparing hundreds of photographic prints. Our thanks also goes to Diane O'Dell for generously sharing her knowledge and technical expertise as a contributing author on spiral CT.

L. C. C.
J. D. L.
V. S. Y-C.

I would like to make a special acknowledgment to my wife, Carolyn, and daughters, Stephanie and Sara, for their understanding, cooperation, and patience while I worked on this book.

J. D. L.

Clinical Computed Tomography for the Technologist

Second Edition

Principles and Instruments of CT

Computed tomography (CT) has become a very important tool in diagnostic medicine, opening up a new world in diagnosis and treatment of disease. Computed tomography uses special detectors to measure the nonabsorbed x-rays passing through a given part of the human anatomy. This information is then sent to a computer to be reconstructed using mathematical equations called algorithms. An image is then displayed on a cathode ray tube (CRT).

The development of CT occurred during the early 1970s because of the work of Godfrey N. Hounsfield. Hounsfield, an engineer, worked for Electrical and Musical Industries (EMI) in London. It was here that he worked on the practical applications of CT scanners. The first clinically usable CT scanner was a head unit installed in 1971 at Atkinson-Morley Hospital in Wimbledon, England.

Advantages of CT over conventional radiography include elimination of superimposed structures, imaging of minute differences in density of anatomical structures and abnormalities, and superior image quality because of considerable reduction of scatter radiation. Because CT scanners utilize a computer, the user also has the ability to manipulate and measure the data. Coronal and sagittal reformations and the ability to measure densities of an anatomical structure are examples of options available because of the use of computer processing.

Third- and Fourth-Generation Scanners

There are two types of CT scanners commonly found in hospitals: third and fourth generation. Advancements in technology have made possible the short scan times and high quality images that these scanners can produce.

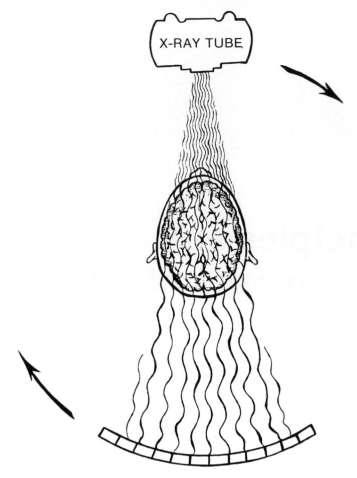

Figure 1.1. Third-generation CT scanner scheme.

Third-generation scanners operate in a manner whereby a fan-shaped x-ray beam and multiple detectors rotate simultaneously around the patient (Fig. 1.1).

Fourth-generation scanners are those wherein a large number of stationary detectors form 360°, and only the fan-shaped x-ray beam rotates around the patient, who is between the x-ray source and the detectors (Fig. 1.2).

Basic CT System

There are three major sections of the basic CT system: (1) the imaging system (gantry, x-ray tube, and detectors); (2) the computer system (develops raw data acquired from detectors and controls the scanner); and (3) display system (operator and viewing console).

IMAGING SYSTEM

The gantry houses the x-ray tube and detectors (Fig. 1.3). It is built so it accommodates the patient in the center of the framework. The circular opening through which the patient moves during scanning is called the gantry aperture.

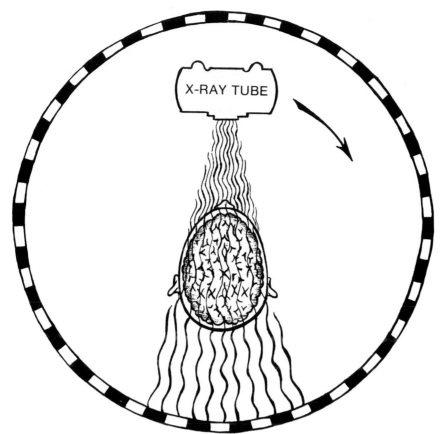

Figure 1.2. Fourth-generation CT scanner scheme.

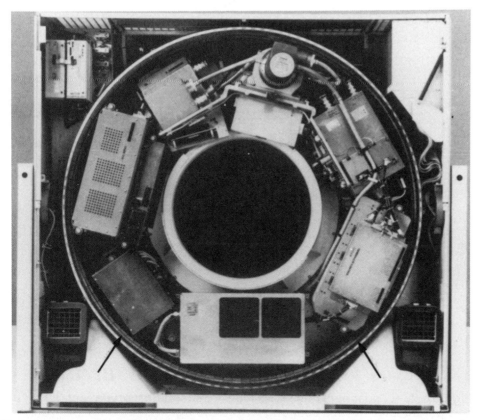

Figure 1.3. Gantry with the front panel removed shows the detector ring *(arrows)*, x-ray tube, and gantry aperture. (Courtesy of Picker International.)

The x-ray tube used in CT has special elements that make it different from a conventional x-ray tube. Tubes used in CT must be able to endure significant stress due to large amounts of exposure made at consistently high milliamperes and kilovolt peaks. Special requirements of CT tubes are higher anode heating capacity. The anode heating capacity in most tubes is typically 1 to 3 million heat units. High-speed rotors are utilized for more efficient heat dissipation.

The requirements of collimation used in CT are no different than in conventional radiography and are used for the same reasons. Collimation reduces patient dose and improves image quality by reducing scatter radiation. There are two collimators used in the CT system: prepatient (x-ray tube) and predetector collimators (Fig. 1.4).

The prepatient (x-ray tube) collimator is located on the tube housing and limits the beam to the patient, thereby limiting patient dose. The predetector collimator limits the x-ray beam to the detector. These collimators are located in front of the detectors to maintain image quality by reducing scatter radiation.

Detectors are a very important part of the CT scanner system, as they gather the information for reconstruction of the image. Basically, the detector is a device that converts x-rays into electrical pulses, which are then fed into a computer for processing.

Detectors must have efficiency to detect x-ray photons, the stability to produce artifact-free images, and a fast response time to detect an x-ray event, recover, and then detect the next one (10).

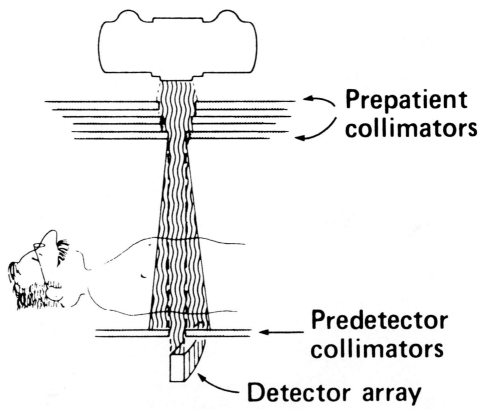

Prepatient collimators

Predetector collimators

Detector array

Figure 1.4. CT scanners utilize two types of collimator: prepatient (x-ray tube) and predetector. (From Bushong SC. *Radiologic Science for the Technologist: Physics, Biology, and Protection.* 5th ed. St. Louis: C.V. Mosby, 1993, with permission.)

There are two basic types of detectors: scintillation and gas ionization.

When initially developed, scintillation detectors were composed of a crystal such as bismuth germinate or sodium iodine coupled to a photomultiplier tube. Currently, the photomultiplier tube has been replaced with solid-state detectors. This type of detector utilizes a crystal such as cadmium tungstate or cesium iodide with a photo diode. Advantages of solid-state detectors are 99% efficiency in converting absorbed photons, low noise, fewer artifacts, and a temperature-stabilized environment. A disadvantage to solid-state detectors is their high cost.

Gas ionization detectors are composed of xenon gas under high pressure. The efficiency of gas detectors is not as good as solid-state detectors. Gas detectors have a photon efficiency of 60% to 93% (1). Even with this poor absorption rate, gas detectors are still used in scanners today, primarily as a result of their low cost.

COMPUTER SYSTEM

The computer, of course, is very important to the scanning system. It is the computer that accepts and processes the data into the image.

Two terms commonly used when discussing computer systems are "hardware" and "software." "Hardware" comprises the physical components of the computer. "Software" is a set of instructions that controls the function of a computer.

There are five fundamental, independent parts to a basic computer: the central processing unit (CPU), memory, input and output devices, and array processor/micro-processor (Fig. 1.5).

The CPU is the heart of the computer. It carries out the main computer functions and conducts the operation of other primary components, for example, causing input and output operations to occur.

The memory unit stores information such as computer programs or instructions.

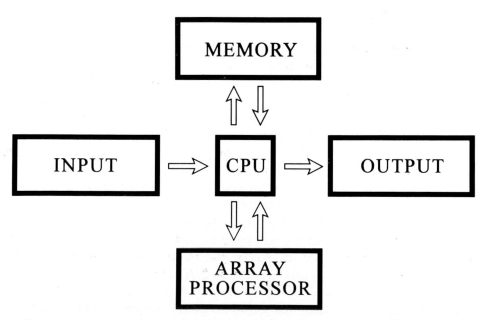

Figure 1.5. Typical components of a computer used in a CT scanner.

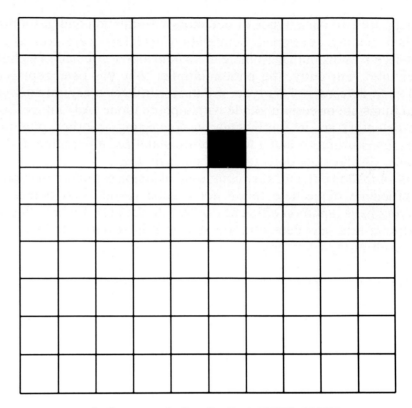

10 x 10 MATRIX

Figure 1.6. A 10 × 10 matrix, which has 100 pixels (picture element). A pixel *(black square)* is a two-dimensional representation of a voxel. As the matrix size increases, the resolution of the CT image improves.

The input device allows the entering of information and instructions to system components. An example of an input device would be a keyboard.

An output device makes the information resulting from processing available for viewing or use. An example of an output device would be a display monitor.

CT scanners use either an array processor or a microprocessor for processing of the scanned data into an image. An advantage to the array processor is its faster speed of image reconstruction. It is this part of the computer that uses the mathematical equation called the algorithm.

Once the image is reconstructed with an algorithm, it is then displayed in a format called a matrix. A matrix is an array of rows and columns of pixels (picture elements) (Fig. 1.6). The pixel is a two-dimensional representation of a voxel (volume element). A voxel is a three-dimensional representation of the amount of x-ray that has been absorbed. The voxel is measured in depth, which is determined by the slice thickness, width, and length, which are results of the pixel size (Fig. 1.7).

The matrix size used in CT will have an impact on the resolution of the image. As the matrix size increases, the image resolution will improve. Commonly used matrix sizes are 256 × 256, 320 × 320, and 512 × 512.

For viewing purposes, each pixel on the display monitor is assigned a shade of gray that corresponds to ranges of CT numbers. These numbers, which are also known as Hounsfield units (HU), range between −1,000

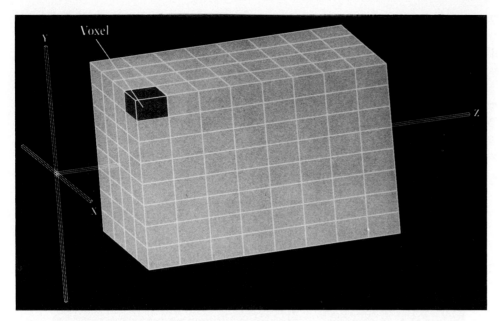

Figure 1.7. A voxel (volume element) is three-dimensional. It is measured in depth (*y*-axis), width (*x*-axis), and length (*z*-axis). (Courtesy Picker International.)

to +1,000, −1,000 representing air, 0 representing water, and +1,000 representing bone. The CT number assigned to each pixel is based on the attenuation coefficient of the object being scanned. The attenuation coefficient is determined by the atomic number of the absorber and photon energy of the x-ray beam.

IMAGE DISPLAY SYSTEM

After the computer has processed the information, we must be able to view and manipulate the data. The equipment that makes up the image display system is the operator's console and the viewing console. It is very difficult to go into great detail about consoles, as they differ so much; these differences make it essential that the technologist study the user's manual for his or her particular machine. All scanners, however, have certain basic functions:

Operator's Console

Essentially, this is where the scanning procedure is controlled. The operator's console is where scanning parameters such as milliamperage, scan time, kilovolt peak, and slice thickness are selected. Patient information (age, sex, name, hospital number) is also entered here to be displayed on what is known as a data page.

Viewing Console

This is where the display and manipulation of the image is done. After the image is processed, it is displayed on the CRT, which is a television-type tube; here the image information is manipulated by control buttons to obtain maximum information. Control buttons on the viewing console allow adjustment of density and contrast and, through software programs, even coronal and sagittal reformations.

Those controls that affect the adjustment of contrast and density are termed the window width ("window") and window level ("level"). The "window" is the range of CT numbers to be viewed, which in essence, controls the contrast of the image. The "level" is the center value of the window width and, in essence, controls the density of the image. For exam-

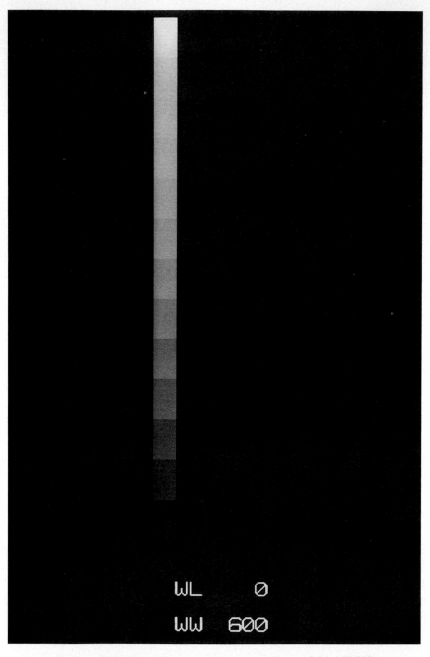

Figure 1.8. Gray scale with a window width *(WW)* of 600 and window level *(WL)* of 0. Only pixels with values between 300 and −300 will appear as shades of gray.

ple, if the window was set at 600 and the level at 0, then those pixels assigned a number above 300 would be represented as pure white and any pixel below −300 would be black. Only pixels with values between 300 and −300 would be displayed in shades of gray (Fig. 1.8).

In summary, the information is sent from the detectors to the computer for processing and then to the viewing console for observation.

References and Suggested Readings

1. Berland LL. *Practical Computer Tomography: technology and techniques*. New York: Raven, 1987.
2. Bushong SC. *Radiologic Science for the Technologist: Physics, Biology, and Protection*. 5th ed. St. Louis: C. V. Mosby, 1993.
3. Droege RT. Quality assurance protocol for CT scanners. *Radiology* 1983;146:244–246.
4. Goodenough DJ, Weaver KE. Factors related to low contrast resolution in CT scanners. *Comput Radiol* 1984;8:297–308.
5. Hounsfield GN. Computed medical imaging: Nobel lecture, December 8, 1979. *J Comput Assist Tomogr* 1980;4:665–674.
6. Hounsfield GN. Computerized transverse axial scanning (tomography). I. Description of system. *Br J Radiol* 1973;46:1016–1022.
7. Judy PF, Swenson RG. Detection of small focal lesions in CT images: effect of reconstruction filters and visual display windows. *Br J Radiol* 1985;58:137–145.
8. McCullough EC. Factors affecting the use of quantitative information from a CT scanner. *Radiology* 1977;124:99–107.
9. McCullough EC, Payne JT. Patient dosage in computed tomography. *Radiology* 1978;129:457–463.
10. Seeram E. *Computed tomography technology*. Philadelphia: W.B. Saunders, 1982.
11. Seeram E. *Computed tomography: physical principles, clinical application, and quality control*. Philadelphia; W.B. Saunders, 1994.
12. Trefler M, Haughton VM. Patient dosage and image quality in computed tomography. *Am J Roentgenol* 1981;137:25–27.

Clinical Considerations for the CT Division and Technologist

CT is an important part of the radiology department, with most hospitals having at least one scanner, and larger hospitals (750 to over 1,000 beds) having two or three units. With CT being an important part of medicine and an increasing number of examinations being done, there are many factors to be considered by the technologist in order to make the CT unit an efficient and progressive area.

Many times, technologists underestimate the importance of communication with the patient. Good patient cooperation can lead to a high-quality examination result, but this cooperation can result only from good communication. Explanations to patients should be brief and in nontechnical terms they can understand. Below is a list of issues the technologist should discuss with the patient before the examination:

1. Briefly explain CT.
2. Describe the examination to be performed (area of body to be covered, examples of what the pictures look like).
3. Give an idea of the length of the procedure.
4. Ask about allergies.
5. If contrast is to be used, explain why and describe its possible effects.
6. Stress that motion is unacceptable and explain what it will do.
7. If necessary, give breathing instructions.
8. Emphasize that even though you are not in the room, you are constantly in visual and verbal contact.

After you have explained the above points, always encourage the patient to ask questions; often there are items they do not completely understand or that you forgot to cover.

Once the examination has begun, periodically step into the room to check on the patient and reassure him or her that you are in visual contact. As

11

Date _____

PROTOCOL FOR HEAD, NECK & SPINE

Patient Name _____ Hosp. No. _____ Age ___ Sex ___

Ward _____ Allergies _____ Bun (10-20) _____ CR (0.7-1.4) _____

CLINICAL INFORMATION:

A. Select type of exam:

( ) Routine brain
( ) Post. fossa/brain
( ) Orbits: ___ coronal ___ axial
( ) Sella: ___ coronal ___ axial
( ) Air cisternogram
( ) Paranasal sinus
( ) Temporal bone
( ) Neck
( ) Spine
( ) Other _____

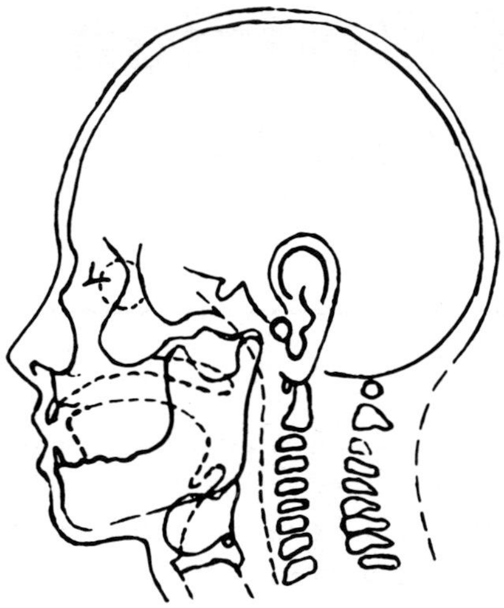

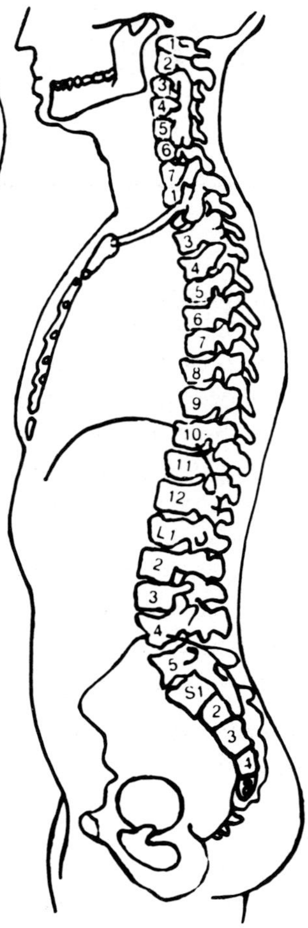

B. Procedure:

( ) with contrast
( ) Drip ___ Bolus ___ Both ___
( ) without/with IV contrast
( ) without IV contrast

C. Scan Instruction:

( ) Thickness/Table index: ___ mm/ ___ mm
( ) Field size: ___ cm.
( ) Dynamic mode _____

D. Comments:

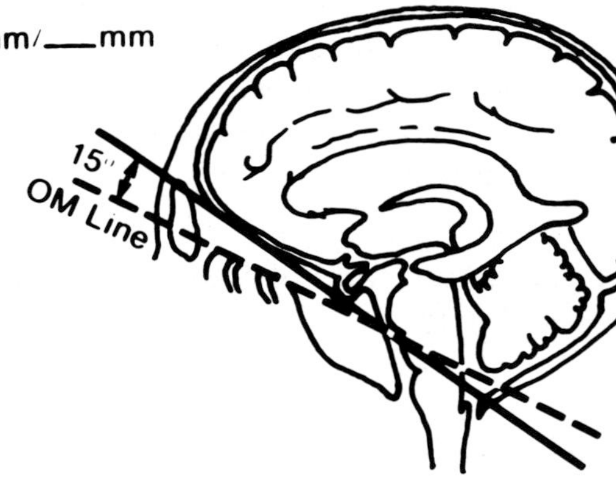

Radiologist _____

CT Technologist _____

A

Figure 2.1. A and **B:** Examples of protocol sheets for use in the CT department.

Date _____

PROTOCOL FOR BODY CT

Patient Name _____ Hosp. No. _____ Age _____ Sex _____

Ward _____ Allergies _____ Bun (10-20) _____ CR (0.7-1.4) _____

CLINICAL INFORMATION

A.   Select type of exam:

( ) Neck   ( ) Chest   ( ) Upper Abdomen   ( ) Abdomen/Pelvis

( ) Pelvis   ( ) Spine   ( ) Extremities

B.   Procedure:

( ) with IV contrast:
( ) __Drip __Bolus __Both
( ) without and with IV contrast
( ) without IV contrast
( ) oral contrast
( ) contrast enema
( ) tampon
( ) air study
( ) other _____

C.   Scan Instruction:

( ) Thickness/Table index: __mm/__mm
( ) Dynamic mode_____
( ) Others _____

D.   Comments:

Radiologist _____

B   CT Technologist _____

technologists, we often think of the CT examination as routine, but to the patient it is an exceptional experience that engenders fear and concern, much of which we can ease by simply being clearly present during the examination.

Often, time is wasted waiting for a radiologist to start intravenous (IV) butterflies or catheters for every examination that needs IV contrast material. This is especially true in large institutions, where a number of examinations are performed daily on two to three machines running a day/evening shift with 75% to 80% of the examinations requiring contrast. Teaching the technologist to start IVs can eliminate this problem and allow a more efficient department. The technologist can be instructed and certified in regard to these techniques and can be made aware of the hazards and reactions that go along with starting IVs and administering contrast material. Most hospitals have medical education committees composed of doctors and nurses who teach these subjects.

The development of protocol sheets (Fig. 2.1A and B) for head and body examinations helps create a more smoothly running department. After a request is received for an examination, the appropriate protocol sheet is attached. These forms are then passed on to the radiologist the day before or the day of the examination for review and checking. After the radiologist selects the examination and procedure that will obtain the most information in regard to the patient's history, the technologist can perform the examination with the checked protocol sheet. These sheets are especially valuable when examinations are performed early in the morning and late in the evening when radiologists are often unavailable for consultation. It is im-

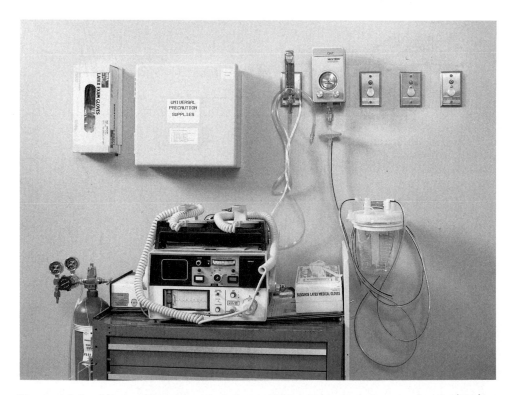

Figure 2.2. All equipment used for patient emergencies and monitoring should be easily accessible and in one specific area of the scanning room. Equipment placed in the room should include a crash cart, suction equipment, blood pressure cuff, oxygen tanks, and cardiac monitor.

portant to have both the radiologist and the technologist initial the protocol sheets in the event of questions.

When medications are given or an unusual incident occurs, the patient's ward or clinic should be called and the circumstances documented on the proper forms. This allows better communication between the department and wards or clinics as well as better patient care.

Technologists should know cardiopulmonary resuscitation (CPR) and be recertified annually. A patient may have a cardiac arrest or drug reaction at any time. There should always be a crash cart available in the department (Fig. 2.2). In addition, a special "contrast reaction tray" containing essential drugs and equipment specifically for contrast reactions should be assembled (see below). The technologists should become familiar with all equipment and supplies and should check regularly to make sure that supplies have not been depleted and the equipment is in good operating condition. The recommended contents of a contrast reaction tray include the following:

Two predrawn epinephrine (1:10,000)	Two syringes (3 cc)
Two predrawn Benadryl (50 mg)	Tape
One predrawn atropine (1.0 mg/10 ml)	Ammonia inhalants
Two ampules atropine (0.4 mg/0.5 ml)	Butterfly needles (19 gauge)
One vial sodium chloride	Butterfly needles (21 gauge)
One bag 5% dextrose	Needles (20 gauge)
One bag 0.9 sodium chloride	Needles (25 gauge)
Two solution administration sets	Abbocath (18 gauge)
One four-way stopcock with extension tube	Abbocath (20 gauge)
One padded tongue blade	Alcohol swabs
Airways, various sizes	Betadine swabs
Two syringes (1 cc)	Tourniquet

Contrast Media Reactions

The use of a positive contrast medium (specifically iodine) plays an important role in helping define pathology and in visualizing vascular structures in CT. Because it is easy to administer and has a high atomic number, iodine is uniquely suited for visualizing structures. However, with its use comes the constant chance of adverse reactions, which can occur after even small amounts (1 ml) have been administered. These reactions are classified into four groups: minor, moderate, major, and fatal.

Minor reactions are those that last briefly and cause the patient some moderate discomfort. Commonly associated symptoms are nausea, vomiting, itching, sweating, and urticaria (hives). Generally no treatment is required with minor reactions.

Moderate reactions are accompanied by a temporary drop in blood pressure, bronchospasms, facial edema, urticaria, and laryngeal edema. Some treatment is required, but moderate reactions are usually not life threatening.

Major reactions are life threatening, and treatment is imperative; without it death can occur. Pulmonary and laryngeal edema along with a prolonged drop in blood pressure, cardiac arrhythmias, and cardiac arrest occur with this type of reaction.

Fatal reactions can occur in all age groups but are seen most frequently in patients over 50 years of age (13).

Before the injection of contrast, there are preventive measures that can be taken to guard against reactions and complications. A detailed history of allergies should be obtained, as patients with a history of allergies are most susceptible to reactions.

If a patient has had a previous reaction to a contrast medium or a history of iodine sensitivity, this is not necessarily a contraindication to its use. A patient who reacts to iodine the first time may not react the second time (14,15). However, extreme caution should be used when injecting these patients.

To help prevent allergic reactions in patients with a history of serious reaction or in those who have a history of multiple allergies, prophylactic therapy is usually practiced. Two types of drug used for this therapy are antihistamines and corticosteroids.

In patients with impaired renal function, iodinated material should be used with caution. Because iodine can act as a toxic agent to the kidneys, it can cause permanent kidney failure in persons already having renal difficulty. (3,4,7,18) Before injection, renal function tests must always be checked. Assays that are of primary concern are creatinine and blood urea nitrogen (BUN). If these are elevated above normal (normal creatinine 0.7–1.4 mg/dl; normal BUN 10–20 mg/dl), the patient's attending physician should be consulted.

If the patient is going to have CT with contrast medium, tests which the patient has already undergone that day must be considered. Often patients have already had tests such as an intravenous pyelogram or another CT that also used intravenous contrast medium. If this situation occurs and the CT is not urgent, it is better to delay it at least 24 hours.

Patients who have multiple myeloma, plasmacytoma, or diabetes should be carefully considered before iodine is used. Because of the nature of their diseases, such patients are especially prone to renal failure.

Seizures, although rare, have been known to occur in patients with primary or secondary metastatic cerebral lesions after administration of contrast medium in cranial CT (6).

Pheochromocytomas are pathological processes that should be recognized before contrast administration. Hypertensive episodes can result from the injection of contrast material, so extreme caution must be exercised in such case if contrast material is necessary.

Since its development, nonionic, low omolar contrast material has seen widespread use as a result of its sixfold reduction of serious reactions (8,11). However, despite this reduction, reactions are not totally eliminated and the opportunity of fatal reactions still exist.

Due to the high cost of nonionic contrast material, which is on the order of approximately 10 times more, its use has not been totally accepted. In most institutions the use of nonionic contrast has been reserved for those patients considered to be at high risk for anophylactoid or chemotoxic reactions.

References and Suggested Readings

1. Bush WH, Mullarkey MF, Webb DR. Adverse reactions to radiographic contrast material. *West J Med* 1980;132:95–9.
2. Bush WH, Swanson DP. Acute reactions to intravascular contrast media: types, risk factors, recognition, and specific treatment. *Am J Roetgenol* 1991;157:1153–1161.
3. Cohen M, Meyers AM, Milne FJ, et al. Acute renal failure after use of radiographic contrast media. *S Afr Med J* 1978;54:662–664.
4. Dawson P. Contrast agent nephrotoxicity: An appraisal. *Br J Radiol* 1985;58:121–124.
5. Elliott LS. Adverse reactions to contrast media: an interview with Elliott Charles Lasser, M. D. *Appl Radiol* 1980;9:63–66.
6. Fischer HW. Occurrence of seizure during cranial computer tomography. *Radiology* 1980;137:563–564.
7. Gale ME, Robbins AH, Hamburger RJ, et al. Renal toxicity of contrast agents: iopamidol, iothalamate, and diatriyoate. *Am J Roetgenol* 1984;143:333–335.
8. Katayama H, Yamaguchi K, Kozuka T, et al. Adverse reaction to ionic and nonionic contrast media. *Radiology* 1990;175:621–628.

9. Lasser EC, Berry CC, Talner LB, et al. Pretreatment with corticosteroids to alleviate reactions to intravenous contrast material. *N Engl J Med* 1987;317:845–849.

10. Pagani JJ, Hayman LA, Bigelow RH, et al. Diazepam prophylaxis of contrast media induced seizures during computed tomography of patients with brain metastases. *Am J Roetgenol* 1983;140:787–792.

11. Palmer FJ. The RACR survey of intravenous contrast media reaction: final report. *Aust Radiol* 1988;32:426–428.

12. Scott WR. Seizures: a reaction to contrast media for computed tomography of the brain. *Radiology* 1980;137:359–361.

13. Shapiro JH. Prevention and management of adverse reactions to intravascular contrast media. ACR Commission on Drugs of the Commission on Public Health, *Am Coll Radiol* 1977;1–3.

14. Shehadi WH. Adverse reactions to intravascularly administered contrast media: a comprehensive study based on a prospective survey. *Radiology* 1975;124:145–152.

15. Shehadi WH. Contrast media adverse reactions: occurrence, recurrence, and distribution patterns. *Radiology* 1982;143:11–17.

16. Shehadi WH, Toniolo G. Adverse reactions to contrast media. *Radiology* 1980;137:299–302.

17. Skucas J. *Radiographic contrast agents.* 2nd ed. Rockville, MD: Aspen Publishers, 1989.

18. Slasky BS, Lenkey JL. Acute renal failure contrast media, and computer tomography. *Urology* 1981;18:309–313.

19. Turner E, Kentor P, Melamed JL, et al. Frequency of anaphylactoid reactions during intravenous urography with radiography contrast media at two different temperatures. *Radiology* 1982;143:327–329.

20. Wood BP, Smith WL. Pulmonary edema in infants following injection of contrast media for urography. *Radiology* 1981;139:377–379.

Brain

Routine Examinations

POSITIONING

Generally, routine head scanning is done with reference to the orbito-meatal line. Scans of the head are performed at a plane that runs at an angle of 15° above this line of reference. Advantages to the use of this plane are: (1) the most information is obtained from the smallest number of slices, thereby reducing scanning time and, more importantly, radiation exposure, particularly to the eyes (28); and (2) artifact is reduced by avoiding as much bone as possible (12,26). Using a lateral localizer for precise positioning, the first slice should start with the foramen magnum in view and then continue until the vertex of the head is seen. During this examination the posterior fossa is not adequately seen in detail; if there is clinical interest in the posterior fossa, a posterior foss (base of skull) examination is recommended.

TECHNIQUE

Slice thicknesses with a range of 8 to 13 mm are commonly used for head scanning. We suggest an 8-mm slice thickness and couch index, which have produced excellent quality examinations consisting of 14 to 16 slices.

To help prevent anatomical asymmetry, the patient's head should always be properly aligned and then immobilized with Velcro straps or tape before any scanning procedure is begun. The use of immobilization straps across the forehead is a constant reminder that movement is unacceptable and that image quality will be degraded by the introduction of motion artifacts. When motion presents a problem in such situations as trauma or in uncoop-erative patients, the same rules apply as in conventional radiography. The milliamperage is increased, and time is decreased. With fourth-generation scanners, exposure times as short as 1 sec have become possible; however, when exposure times are decreased, contrast resolution is sacrificed.

Posterior Fossa

POSITIONING

Positioning for a posterior fossa examination is identical to that for a brain examination. Scanning is done in the same plane, with the first slice having the foramen magnum in view. Scanning then continues upward to the level at which the tentorium cerebelli comes together, approximately even with the bodies of the lateral ventricles. At this level, the study is complete if no lesions are seen.

TECHNIQUE

Because of the anatomical detail located in the posterior fossa, smaller thickness and couch indexing are necessary. A 4-5 mm slice thickness and couch index are frequently used to evaluate anatomical structures in examinations consisting of 11 to 13 slices.

Contrast Enhancement

IODINE

Intravenous (IV) contrast medium plays an important part in determining and characterizing cranial pathology. Its use can help answer questions on such findings as mass effect, edema, and hypo- or hyperdense areas present on unenhanced scans. The use of IV contrast medium is particularly important during examinations for suspicion of brain lesions. Because many of these lesions are enhanced through a phenomenon called the "blood-brain barrier," iodine often characterizes lesions by the way they enhance.

The choice of performing the examination with or without contrast enhancement or performing two separate examinations (the first one without, the second with) depends on the clinical history and the physical examination. Table 4.1 summarizes our suggestions regarding the use of iodine.

IODINE CONTRAST ENHANCEMENT TECHNIQUES

The movement of contrast medium in the brain differs significantly from that in the body. Instead of contrast going from an intravascular space to an extravascular space, as in the body, it must go through one additional step in the brain.

Inside the brain there is an intact blood-brain barrier that precedes the extravasation of contrast medium to the extravascular space. Because most of the abnormal enhancement of a tumor results from passage of contrast medium into the extracellular compartment of a lesion through a deficiency in the blood-brain barrier, enhancement may occur slowly (2). Because structural and vascular detail become increased by high levels of intravascular contrast medium, any good method of contrast administration provides a maintained moderate plasma concentration of the contrast medium before scanning to allow equilibration with the extravascular com-

Table 4.1. *Suggestions for the use of iodinated contrast enhancement*

Without IV contrast	With IV contrast	Without and with IV contrast
Intracranial hemorrhage	Primary and secondary brain tumors	Cerebral vascular accident
Traumatic hemorrhage	Brain abscess and infection (e.g., herpes, encephalitis)	Arteriovenous malformation
Motor vehicle accident	Recurrent brain tumors	Aneurysm and other vascular lesions
Fall	Sellar lesions	Posterior fossa lesions
Gunshot wound	Nonspecific (suspect organic lesion as cause)	
Immediate postoperative procedure	Dementia	
Nontraumatic hemorrhage	Headache	
Subarachnoid hemorrhage	Seizures	
Hypertensive hemorrhage		
Anticoagulant therapy		
Iodine allergy		
Poor renal function		
Hydrocephalus		

partment and a high plasma concentration during scanning to promote improved imaging of vascular structures (2).

Methods commonly used for contrast enhancement in cranial CT are: (1) drip infusion; (2) bolus injection only; (3) drip infusion, then bolus injection; and (4) bolus injection, then drip infusion.

Drip Infusion

Use of a rapid drip infusion of 150 ml of contrast medium usually gives satisfactory enhancement of the cranial parenchyma and vasculature. A major problem with the drip infusion technique is the slow rise in plasma iodine concentration owing to intermittent contrast flow.

Bolus Injection Only

A bolus injection gives an immediately elevated plasma iodine concentration that is effective for 2 to 3 min. This technique is commonly used with rapid scanning when there is a primary area of interest. Because the effective plasma iodine level lasts a short time, it should not be used in routine examinations.

Drip Infusion, Then Bolus Injection

In the drip infusion/bolus injection technique (Fig. 4.1) a rapid drip infusion of 150 ml of contrast medium is used to saturate the tissue. Then immediately before scanning begins, a bolus injection of 30 ml is administered to obtain a high plasma iodine concentration that lasts a short time

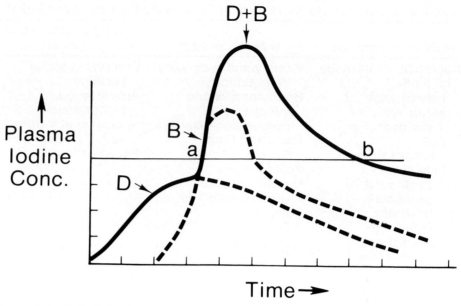

Figure 4.1. Drip infusion followed by a bolus injection. After a standard drip infusion *(curve D),* a bolus of contrast medium *(curve B)* results in a high "peak" iodine concentration *(D + B)* that lasts a short time; during this time *(a–b* line) the scan is obtained. (Modified from Burman and Rosenbaum. *Radiol Clin North Am* 1982;20:15–22; with permission.)

(Fig. 4.1, *a–b* line). During the period of high iodine concentration a series of images are obtained. Due to the high plasma iodine concentration, there is good demonstration of vascular structures. This technique also aids in the enhancement at pathological sites because of extravasation past the blood-brain barrier from the initial drip infusion (2).

Bolus Injection, Then Drip Infusion

A bolus may be used to obtain an initial elevated plasma iodine value and then be followed by a rapid drip to help maintain the plasma iodine concentration throughout the examination (Fig. 4.2). This technique has been found to provide accurate diagnostic information, and it is also convenient.

Because of its high initial iodine load, which can be maintained by rapid infusion after the bolus, the bolus injection/drip infusion technique is, in our experience, the optimal technique for contrast during cranial CT. Iodine doses ranging from 51 to 74 g have been found to provide a good diagnostic study and accurate information (23). We suggest a 30-ml bolus of contrast followed by a 150-ml bottle of contrast medium infused at a rapid rate. The scan begins when the bottle is half-empty.

METRIZAMIDE

Metrizamide often plays an important role in the diagnosis of cranial lesions, congenital anomalies, and posttraumatic fistulas. That it is water-soluble, mixes well with cerebrospinal fluid (CSF), and has a low viscosity

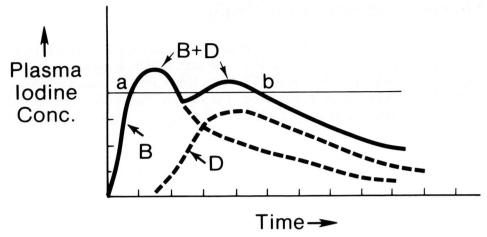

Figure 4.2. Bolus injection followed by drip infusion. The curved line *B + D* illustrates the summation of the drip infusion curve and bolus injection curve. Optimal opacification is evenly maintained for most of the examination. (Modified from Burman and Rosenbaum. *Radiol Clin North Am* 1982;20:15–22; with permission.)

make it possible to get distinct visualization of the cisterns, subarachnoid space, and brainstem, which is outlined by surrounding cisterns. This distinct visualization makes it easier to determine normal shape, size, and position of these structures. It is commonly used to evaluate the brainstem for tumors, Chiari malformations, and localization of CSF leaks (8,9, 20,25).

Because metrizamide gives excellent visualization of the cisterns and outlines the brainstem, its use with CT is often best for brainstem tumors. Small suspected lesions that do not show to satisfaction with intravenous contrast can usually be diagnosed by their compression or displacement by metrizamide-opacified structures.

Cerebellar tonsil herniation and spinal cord widening are most easily identified with metrizamide and CT, making identification of congenital craniocerebral anomalies such as Chiari malformations much simpler.

Metrizamide CT cisternography has also simplified anatomical location of CSF leaks. Because metrizamide mixes well with CSF, CSF leaks due to traumatic injury causing a fistula between the subarachnoid space and paranasal sinuses or middle ear can be accurately located.

Magnetic resonance imaging (MRI) has become the optimal imaging modality for evaluating the brainstem for tumors and Chiari malformations. Metrizamide CT is reserved for patients who cannot undergo or tolerate MRI.

Bone Levels

Bone levels add greatly to information regarding fractures and pathological conditions of the head. With their aid, skull fractures and bone changes resulting from metastatic lesions are quite easily seen. When examinations are done on patients suspected of having bone destruction, these levels should be included as part of the examination.

Normal Anatomy of the Brain

The following series of brain images (Figs. 4.3 through 4.11) were obtained at 80 mA, an exposure time of 4.6 sec, a 360° scan angle, and a couch index and slice thickness of 8 mm. For contrast enhancement a bolus/drip infusion method was used. Figs. 4.3A and 4.4A were photographed at a bone technique for visualization of bony structures.

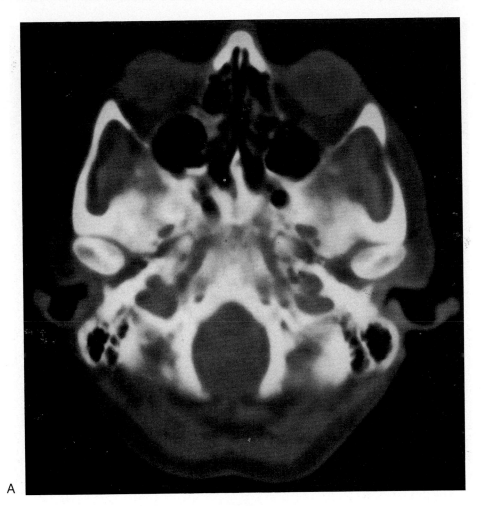

A

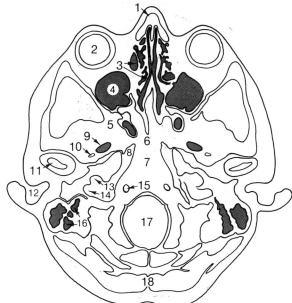

B

Figure 4.3. A,B: *(1)* Nasal bone. *(2)* Globe. *(3)* Ethmoid sinus. *(4)* Maxillary sinus. *(5)* Greater wing of sphenoid bone. *(6)* Body of sphenoid bone. *(7)* Clivus. *(8)* Foramen lacerum. *(9)* Foramen ovale. *(10)* Foramen spinosum. *(11)* Mandibular condyle. *(12)* External auditory canal. *(13)* Internal carotid canal. *(14)* Internal jugular foramen. *(15)* Hypoglossal canal. *(16)* Mastoid air cells. *(17)* Medulla oblongata. *(18)* Ligamentum nuchae.

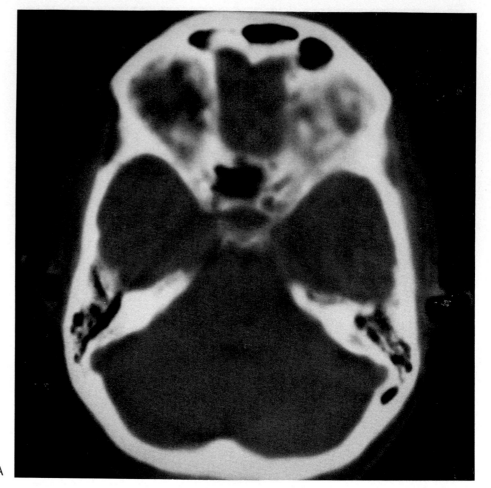

A

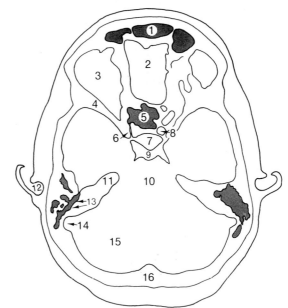

B

Figure 4.4. A and **B:** *(1)* Frontal sinus. *(2)* Frontal lobe. *(3)* Roof of orbit. *(4)* Greater wing of sphenoid bone. *(5)* Sphenoid sinus. *(6)* Anterior clinoids. *(7)* Pituitary fossa. *(8)* Internal carotid canal. *(9)* Dorsum sella. *(10)* Pons. *(11)* Petrous bone. *(12)* External auditory canal. *(13)* Mastoid air cells. *(14)* Sigmoid sinus area. *(15)* Cerebellar hemisphere. *(16)* Internal occipital crest.

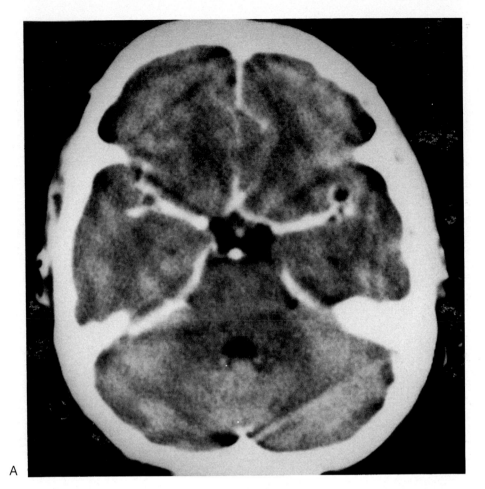

A

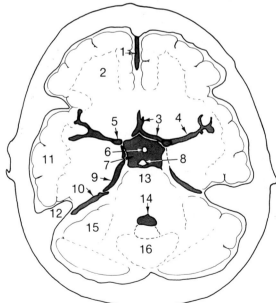

B

Figure 4.5. A and **B:** *(1)* Falx cerebri. *(2)* Frontal lobe. *(3)* Anterior cerebral artery. *(4)* Middle cerebral artery. *(5)* Internal carotid artery. *(6)* Infundibulum of pituitary gland (stalk). *(7)* Suprasellar cistern. *(8)* Basilar artery. *(9)* Posterior cerebral artery. *(10)* Tentorium cerebelli. *(11)* Temporal lobe. *(12)* Petrous bone. *(13)* Pons. *(14)* Fourth ventricle. *(15)* Cerebellar hemisphere. *(16)* Cerebellar vermis.

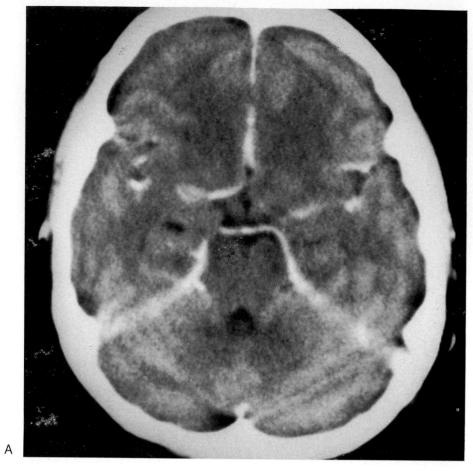

A

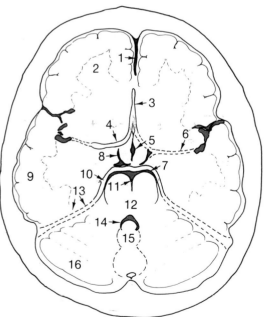

B

Figure 4.6. A and **B:** *(1)* Falx cerebri. *(2)* Frontal lobe. *(3)* Anterior cerebral artery. *(4)* Middle cerebral artery. *(5)* Inferior recess of third ventricle. *(6)* Middle cerebral artery. *(7)* Cerebellopontine angle cistern. *(8)* Suprasellar cistern. *(9)* Temporal lobe. *(10)* Posterior cerebral artery. *(11)* Interpeduncular cistern. *(12)* Pons. *(13)* Tentorium cerebelli. *(14)* Fourth ventricle. *(15)* Cerebellar vermis. *(16)* Cerebellar hemisphere.

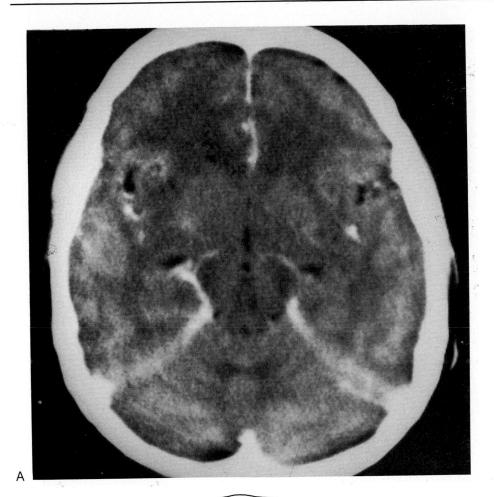

A

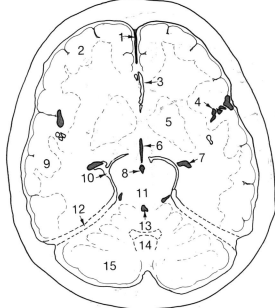

B

Figure 4.7. A and **B:** *(1)* Falx cerebri. *(2)* Frontal lobe. *(3)* Anterior cerebral artery. *(4)* Sylvian fissure. *(5)* Putamen. *(6)* Third ventricle. *(7)* Choroidal fissure. *(8)* Interpeduncular cistern. *(9)* Temporal lobe. *(10)* Posterior cerebral artery. *(11)* Midbrain. *(12)* Tentorium cerebelli. *(13)* Cerebral aqueduct. *(14)* Cerebellar vermis. *(15)* Cerebellar hemisphere.

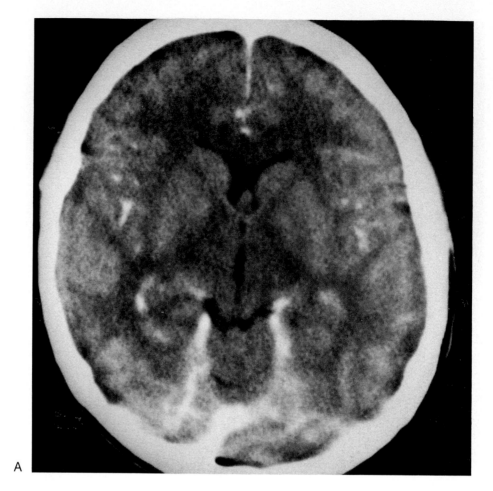

A

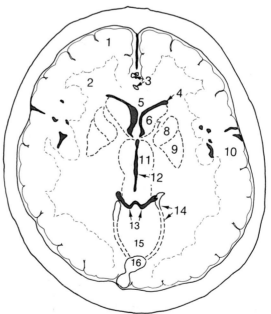

B

Figure 4.8. A and **B:** *(1)* Gray matter. *(2)* White matter. *(3)* Anterior cerebral artery branches. *(4)* Anterior horns of lateral ventricles. *(5)* Genu of corpus callosum. *(6)* Head of caudate nucleus. *(7)* Anterior limb of internal capsule. *(8)* Putamen. *(9)* Globus pallidus. *(10)* Temporal lobe. *(11)* Hypothalamus. *(12)* Third ventricle. *(13)* Quadrigeminal cistern. *(14)* Tentorium cerebelli. *(15)* Cerebellar vermis. *(16)* Torcular herophili.

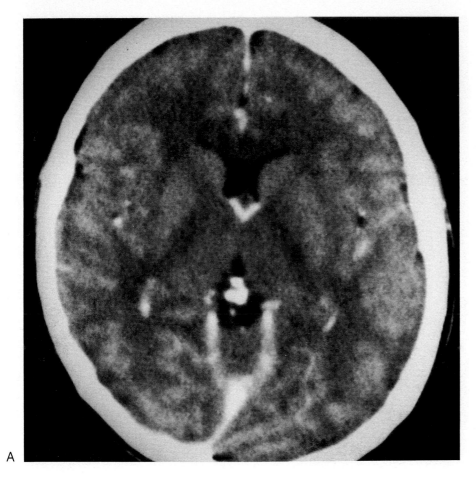

A

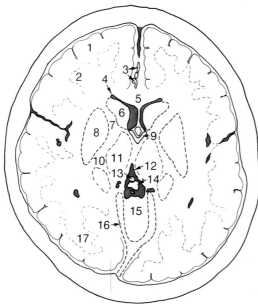

B

Figure 4.9. A and **B:** *(1)* Gray matter. *(2)* White matter. *(3)* Anterior cerebral artery branches. *(4)* Anterior horns of lateral ventricles. *(5)* Genu of corpus callosum. *(6)* Head of caudate nucleus. *(7)* Anterior limb of internal capsule. *(8)* Putamen. *(9)* Thalamostrate vein. *(10)* Posterior limb of internal capsule. *(11)* Thalamus. *(12)* Third ventricle. *(13)* Habenular commissure. *(14)* Pineal body. *(15)* Cerebellar vermis. *(16)* Tentorium cerebelli. *(17)* Occipital lobe.

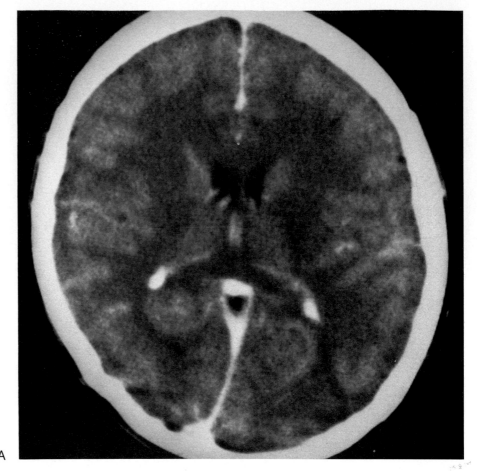

A

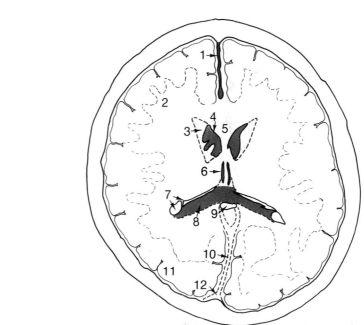

B

Figure 4.10. A and **B:** *(1)* Falx cerebri. *(2)* Frontal lobe. *(3)* Head of caudate nucleus. *(4)* Anterior horns of the lateral ventricles. *(5)* Genu of corpus callosum. *(6)* Internal cerebral veins. *(7)* Choroid plexus of lateral ventricle. *(8)* Lateral ventricle. *(9)* Vein of Galen. *(10)* Straight sinus. *(11)* Occipital lobe. *(12)* Superior sagittal sinus.

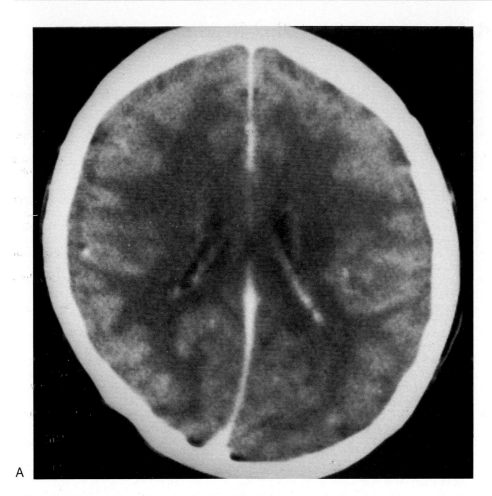

A

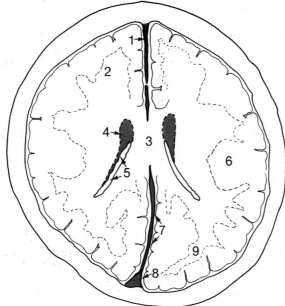

B

Figure 4.11. A and **B:** *(1)* Falx cerebri (anterior). *(2)* Frontal lobe. *(3)* Corpus callosum. *(4)* Lateral ventricle. *(5)* Choroid plexus of lateral ventricle. *(6)* Parietal lobe. *(7)* Falx cerebri (posterior). *(8)* Superior sagittal sinus. *(9)* Occipital lobe.

References and Suggested Readings

1. Bradac GB, Schramm J, Grumme T, et al. CT of the base of the skull. *Neuroradiology* 1978;17:1–5.
2. Burman S, Rosenbaum AE. Rationale and techniques for intravenous enhancement in computed tomography. *Radiol Clin North Am* 1982;20:15–22.
3. Burrows EH. Surface enhancement of the brain. *Clin Radiol* 1985;36:233–239.
4. Catell WR, Kerlsey F, Spencer AG, et al. Excretion urography: factors determining the excretion of Hypaque. *Br J Radiol* 1967;40:561–580.
5. Chakeres DW, Kapila A. Brainstem and related structures: normal CT anatomy using direct longitudinal scanning with metrizamide cisternography. *Radiology* 1983;149:709–715.
6. Claussenb CD, Bansjer D, Pfretsyschner C, et al. Bolus geometry and dynamics after intravenous contrast medium injection. *Radiology* 1984;153:365–368.
7. Huckman MS, Russel EJ. Selecting an optimal plane for CT examination of the base of the skull. *Am J Neuroradiol* 1984;333–334.
8. Ghoshhajra K. Metrizamide CT cisternography in the diagnosis and localization of cerebrospinal fluid rhinorrhea. *J Comput Assist Tomogr* 1980;4:306–310.
9. Glanz S, Geehr RB, Duncan CC, Piepmeier JM. Metrizamide-enhanced CT for evaluation of brainstem tumors. *Am J Roentgenol* 1980;134:821–824.
10. Hammerschlag SB, Wolpert SM, Carter BL. Computed tomography of the skull base. *J Comput Assist Tomogr* 1977;1:75.
11. Hryshko FG, Deeb ZL. Computed tomography in acute head injuries. *J Comput Tomogr* 1983;7:331–344.
12. Kieffer SA, Heitzman ER. *An atlas of cross-sectional anatomy: computed tomography, ultrasound, radiography, gross anatomy.* Hagerstown, MD: Harper & Row, 1979.
13. Kobayashi M, Saito Y, Miyashita T, et al. Cisternography of the posterior fossa with metrizamide. *Radiology* 1981;141:819–821.
14. Latchaw RE, Gold LHA, Tourje EJ. A protocol for the use of contrast enhancement in cranial computed tomography. *Radiology* 1978;126:681–687.
15. Lee SH, Rao KCVG. *Cranial computed tomography.* New York: McGraw-Hill Book Co., 1983.
16. Lennington BR, Laster DW, Moody DM, et al. Pre-enhancement ring density in resolving intracerebral hematomas. *Comput Tomogr* 1979;3:105–109.
17. Lin JP. Computed tomography of the head in adults. *Postgrad Med* 1976;2:113–118.
18. Martin JB, Reichlin S, Brown GM. *Clinical neuroendocrinology.* Philadelphia: Davis, 1977;240–243.
19. Mawad ME, Silver AJ, Hilal SK. Computed tomography of the brain stem with intrathecal metrizamide. I. The normal brainstem. *Am J Roetgenol* 1983;140:553–563.
20. Mawad ME, Silver AJ, Hilal SK. Computed tomography of the brain stem with intrathecal metrizamide. II. Lesions in and around the brain stem. *Am J Roetgenol* 1983;140:553–563.
21. Newhouse J. Fluid compartment distribution of intravenous iothalamate in the dog. *Invest Radiol* 1977;12:364–367.
22. Podlas H. Diagnosis of posterior fossa lesions by computed tomography. *Appl Radiol* 1980;9:26–35.
23. Raininko R, Majurin ML, Virtama P, et al. Value of high contrast medium dose in brain CT. *J Comput Assist Tomogr* 1982;6:54–57.
24. Rieth KG, Schwartz FT, Davis DO. Acute isodense epidural hematoma on computed tomography. *J Comput Assist Tomogr* 1979;3:691–693.
25. Steele JR, Hoffman JC. Brainstem evaluation with CT cisternography. *Am J Roetgenol* 1981;136:287–292.
26. Valk J. *Computed tomography and cerebral infarctions.* New York: Raven Press, 1980.
27. Weisburg LA. The role of CT in the evaluation of patients with intracranial CNS infections—inflammatory disorders. *Comput Radiol* 1984;8:29–36.
28. Yeoman LJ, Howath L, Britten A, et al. Gantry angulation in brain CT: dosage implications, effect on posterior fossa artifacts, and current international practice. *Radiology* 1992;184:113–116.
29. Zimmerman RD, Danziger A. Extracerebral trauma. *Radiol Clin North Am* 1982;20:105–120.

Sella

Positioning

CORONAL PROJECTION

Generally, sella examinations are done in the coronal projection. This projection gives excellent visualization of the pituitary gland (especially its thickness), sellar floor, and suprasellar cistern. Also better defined in this projection are the superior and inferior margins of a lesion, its origin, and its relationship to surrounding structures (7,15,16). These characteristics plus the fact that small lesions (less than 1 cm) such as microadenomas can be overlooked by partial volume averaging from bone and suprasellar cistern in the axial position make coronal positioning the optimal method (15).

Before a coronal examination is started, all dentures and partial plates are removed to help eliminate metal-induced artifact.

For coronal projections, the patient is usually placed in the supine position with a pillow under the buttocks and a pad under the shoulders to help obtain maximum hyperextension of the neck (Fig. 5.1). The head is dropped back so the vertex rests on a head support. A lateral localizer is taken, and the scanning plane is positioned so it runs perpendicular to the floor of the sella with the first slice beginning on the anterior clinoids. Scanning ends at the dorsum sella. Since filling-induced artifact is the main problem with coronal scanning, maximum hyperextension of the head should be optimized so that the sella and teeth are not superimposed. The scanning gantry may also need to be tilted so dental fillings are avoided.

PRONE POSITION

The coronal projection can also be obtained with the patient in the prone position. In this position the patient is placed on his or her stomach with

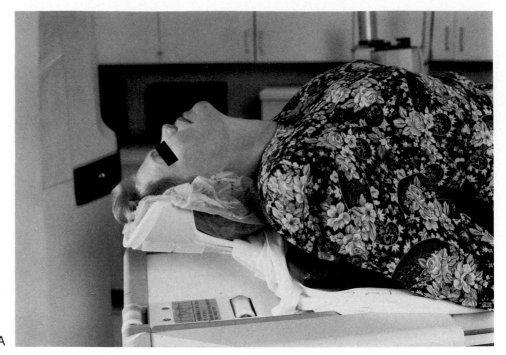

A

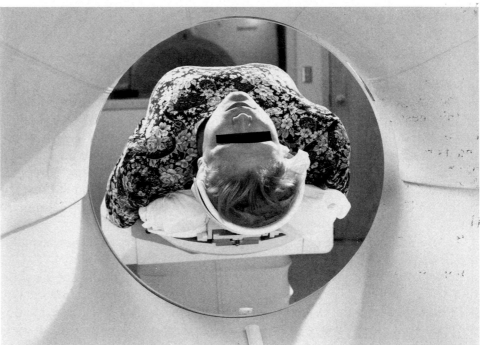

B

Figure 5.1. Supine coronal position. **(A)** Building the patient's shoulders up helps obtain maximum hyperextension of the neck. The surgical cap on the patient's head helps eliminate artifact caused by hair that is out of the scanning field. **(B)** View of the patient from behind the scanning gantry.

arms at the sides. The neck is then extended with the head resting on the chin (Fig. 5.2).

Use of either the prone or the supine position for coronal views varies among institutions. Generally, the patient can be immobilized more completely and hyperextension of the neck is easier to achieve in the supine position.

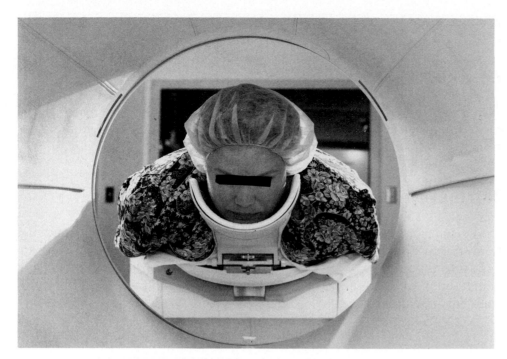

Figure 5.2. Patient in the prone coronal position.

Both of these positions are difficult for the patient to maintain, and there are many times when they cannot be used. If it appears that the patient cannot assume the position and image quality will be degraded by motion and asymmetry, axial positions should be utilized.

It is important to use the position that yields the most information in each situation.

AXIAL POSITION

If maximal hyperextension is not achievable, and dental fillings will obscure slice detail, the axial position must be used. To position for axial projections, the patient is placed supine on a head-holder with the infraorbitomeatal line perpendicular to the room floor. A lateral localizer is taken, with the first slice beginning at and perpendicular to the floor of the sella. Once the area of the lateral ventricles is reached, the study is terminated if no extension of the lesion is seen.

Technique

Because a normal sella is a miniature structure with thin bone, accurate CT evaluation requires a detailed scanning mode. Thin, adjacent sections should be used in order to avoid substandard images due to partial volume effect. A 2-mm slice thickness and couch index will give excellent detail.

To make a complete examination of the sella, multiplanar reformations are done in coronal and sagittal planes. With coronal and sagittal reformations more dimensions are added that can help distinguish the extent and relationship of abnormal pathology to surrounding structures. Suggested routine reconstruction is midline at the level of the anterior clinoids (Fig. 5.7).

CONTRAST ENHANCEMENT

Sella examinations are routinely performed with contrast material, as most pituitary and parasellar masses enhance significantly after administration of intravenous contrast (see Contrast Enhancement; Chapter 4).

Normal Anatomy of the Sella

The sellar images in Figs. 5.3 through 5.6 were performed with the patient in the supine coronal position. Scanning was done using 65 mA, an exposure time of 9.3 sec, and a 360° scan angle. The slice thickness and couch index were 2 mm. A bolus/drip infusion method was used for contrast enhancement.

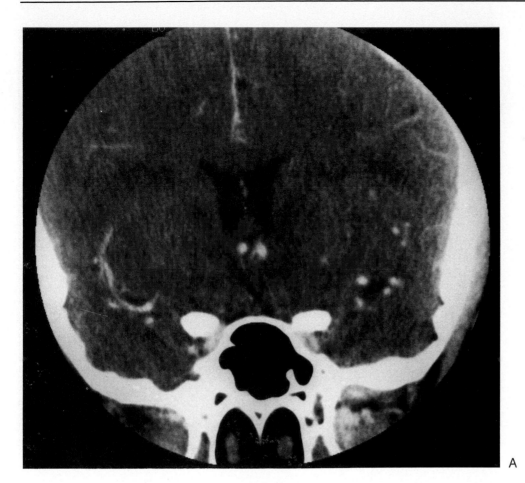

A

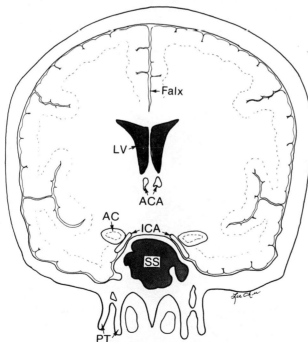

B

Figure 5.3. A and **B:** This section at the level of the anterior clinoids *(AC)* shows the internal carotid arteries *(ICA)* emerging into the cranium between the sphenoid sinus *(SS)* and anterior clinoids. A segment of the anterior cerebral artery *(ACA)* is seen inferior to the anterior horns of the lateral ventricles *(LV)*. *PT,* pterygoids.

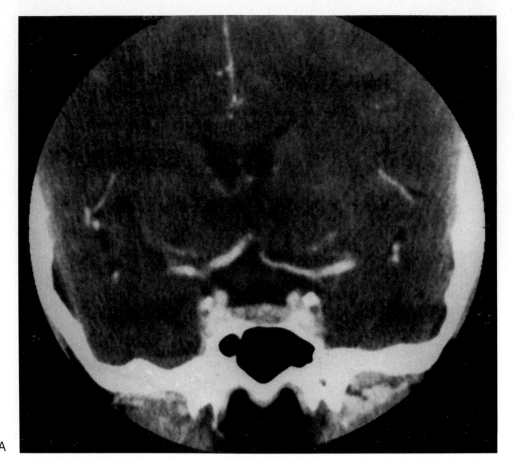

A

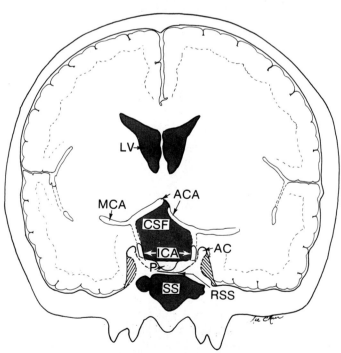

B

Figure 5.4. A and **B:** In this section the anterior cerebral artery *(ACA)* and middle cerebral artery *(MCA)* are seen branching off the internal carotid artery *(ICA)*. The pituitary gland *(P)* is outlined by cerebrospinal fluid *(CSF)* in the suprasellar cistern superiorly and inferiorly by the roof of the sphenoid sinus *(RSS* = floor of sella). *AC,* anterior clinoids. *LV,* lateral ventricles. *SS,* sphenoid sinus.

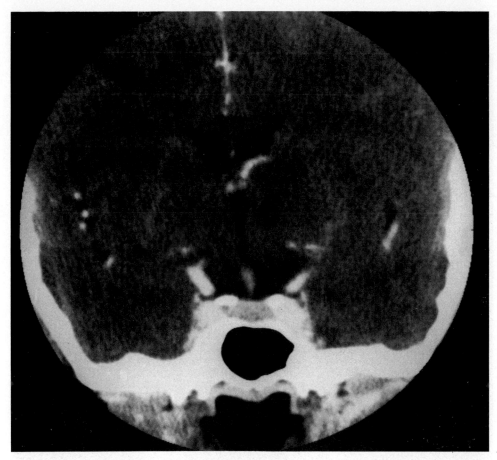

A

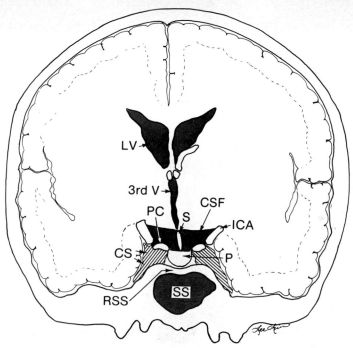

B

Figure 5.5. A and **B:** This section at the body of the lateral ventricles *(LV)* and anterior portion of the third ventricle *(3rd V)* clearly shows the stalk *(S)* (also known as the infundibulum) and the pituitary gland *(P)*, outlined by suprasellar cerebrospinal fluid *(CSF)*. Note the homogeneous enhancement bilaterally surrounding the pituitary gland *(P)*. This represents the cavernous sinus *(CS)*. The III, IV, V, and VI cranial nerves and internal carotid arteries are located within the cavernous sinus. The tips of the posterior clinoids *(PC)* are also seen. *RSS*, roof of sphenoid sinus (= floor of sella). *SS*, sphenoid sinus.

43

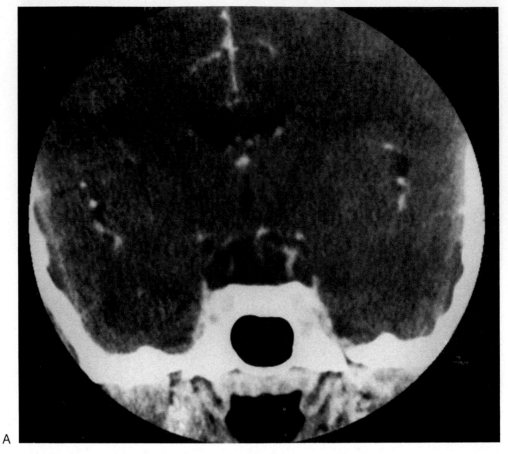

A

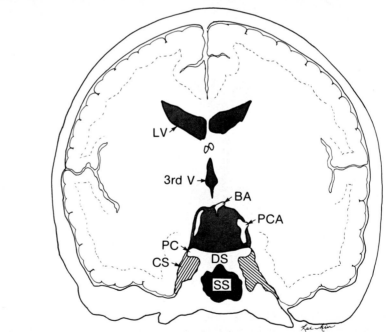

B

Figure 5.6. A and **B:** In this section the dorsum sella *(DS)*, posterior clinoids *(PC)*, and cavernous sinus *(CS)* are well visualized. The pituitary gland is no longer seen. Note that portions of the posterior cerebral artery *(PCA)* and basilar artery *(BA)* are seen. *LV,* lateral ventricles. *SS,* sphenoid sinus. *3rd V,* third ventricle.

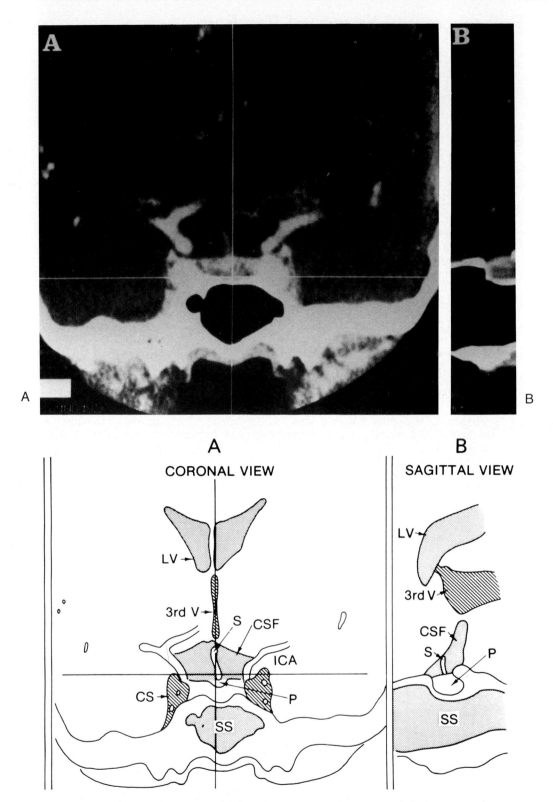

Figure 5.7. A and **B:** Reformation from a coronal view *(A)* demonstrates a sagittal view *(B)* of the pituitary gland *(P)* and surrounding structures. *CSF*, cerebrospinal fluid. *LV*, lateral ventricle. *3rd V*, third ventricle. *S*, stalk or infundibulum. *SS*, sphenoid sinus. *CS*, cavernous sinus. *ICA*, internal carotid artery.

References and Suggested Readings

1. Bilaniuk LT, Moshang T, Cara J, et al. Pituitary enlargement mimicking pituitary tumor. *J Neurosurg* 1985;63:39–42.
2. Earnest F, McCullough EC, Frank DA. Fact or artifact: an analysis of artifact in high-resolution computed tomographic scanning of the sella. *Neuroradiology* 1981;140:109–113.
3. Elster AD. Modern imaging of the pituitary. *Radiology* 1993;187:1–14.
4. Fong TC, Johns RD, Long M, Myles ST. CT of pituitary abscess. *Am J Roetgenol* 1985;1141–1142.
5. Guy RL, Benn JJ, Ayers AB, et al. Comparison of CT and MRI in the assessment of the pituitary and parasellar region. *Clin Radiol* 1991;43:156–161.
6. Kricheff II. The radiologic diagnosis of pituitary adenoma. *Radiology* 1979;131:263–265.
7. Levine HL, Kleefield J, Rao KCVG. The base of the skull. In: *Cranial computed tomography*. New York: McGraw-Hill Book Co., 1983, 372–459.
8. Lundin P, Bergstrom K. Thuomas KA, et al. Comparison MR imaging and CT in pituitary maroadenomas. *Acta Radiol* 1991;32:189–196.
9. Mass S, Norman D, Newton TH. Coronal computed tomography: indications and accuracy. *Am J Roetgenol* 1978;131:875–879.
10. Peyster RG, Hoover ED. CT of the normal pituitary stalk. *Am J Neuroradiol* 1984;4:45–47.
11. Peyster RG, Hoover ED. CT of the abnormal pituitary stalk. *Am J Neuroradiol* 1984;4:49–52.
12. Robertson HJ, Rose A, Ehmi B, et al. Trends in the radiological study of pituitary adenoma. *Neuroradiology* 1981;21:75–78.
13. Swartz JD, Russell KB, Basile BA, et al. High resolution computed tomography of the intrasellar contents: normal, near normal and abnormal. *Radiographics* 1983;3:228–247.
14. Syvertsen A, Haughton VM, Williams AL, Cusick JF. The computed tomographic appearance of the normal pituitary gland and pituitary microadenomas. *Radiology* 1979;133:385–391.
15. Taylor S. High resolution computed tomography of the sella. *Radiol Clin North Am* 1982;20:207–236.
16. Wolfman NT, Boehnke M. The use of coronal sections in evaluation lesions of the sellar and parasellar regions. *J Comput Assist Tomogr* 1978;2:308–313.
17. Wolpert SM. Radiology of pituitary adenomas. *Semin Roetengol* 1984;19:53–69.

6

Orbit

Positioning and Techniques

Routine orbital examinations may be performed in one of two ways: (1) in the axial plane only, using thin sectioning; or (2) by combining axial scanning with direct coronal scanning, employing thicker sections.

AXIAL PLANE ONLY

With the patient in the axial position, the head is placed so the infraorbitomeatal line is perpendicular to the floor. A lateral localizer is used, and the scanning plane is positioned so slices are taken parallel to the orbit floor.

Because optic nerves run in an uneven course, it is important to instruct patients to direct their eyes upward. With upward gaze, as the anterior part of the globe rotates upward, the optic nerve is displaced downward with the posterior globe. The position straightens most of the nerve except the most anterior part, where it curves upward to attach to the globe (5). An object is provided for the patient to focus on by placing a 0.75-inch-diameter self-stick label on the front, top portion of the gantry aperture.

When only the axial plane is used, thin sections (1.5 to 3 mm) are implemented. Thin sectioning improves the definition of orbital structures, helps eliminate partial volume averaging, and gives improved multiplanar reformations.

Good multiplanar reformations are important when only axial sections are taken (12). Axial sections alone cannot always define the extent and relationship of abnormal pathology to surrounding structures. With coronal and sagittal reformations, two more dimensions are added to gain a better perspective of lesions and diseases. To achieve high-quality and multiplanar reformations, motion by the patient must be minimal.

There are five areas suggested for reformations (see Fig. 6.5): (1) lens, (2) midglobe, (3) optic disc, (4) mid-optic nerve, and (5) orbital fissure.

These reformations are routinely performed. When a lesion is found, reformations are made directly in the affected area to better define its extent and relationship to surrounding structures.

COMBINED AXIAL AND DIRECT CORONAL SCANNING

Both axial and direct coronal positions may be used, with the scanning usually done at a slice thickness and couch index of 5 mm. The patient may be positioned for the coronal projection using either the prone or the supine method. To avoid artifacts from dental fillings when performing coronal scanning, the patient's head must be extended to approximately 65° (3,4). With this extension and slight angulation of the gantry, good-quality images can easily be obtained.

Procedures done using this method will result in a shorter examination time. Moreover, because the direct coronal position is utilized, orbital and paraorbital anatomy is seen in a different perspective without loss of detail.

Contrast Enhancement

The choice of contrast enhancement is indicated by the clinical and physical history. Although contrast is often not indicated, there is always a high level of inherent contrast provided by orbital fat. When orbital neoplasms and vascular abnormalities are in question, contrast enhancement can prove helpful.

Normal Anatomy of the Orbit

The following orbital images (Figs. 6.1 through 6.5) were obtained using 65 mA, an exposure time of 6.2 sec, and a scan angle of 360°. A slice thickness and couch index of 3 mm was used. For contrast enhancement, a bolus/drip infusion method was used.

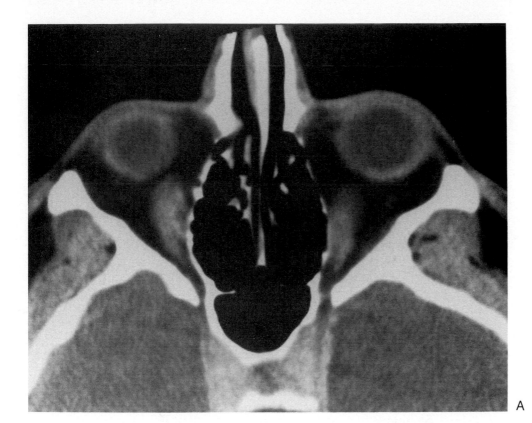

Section A

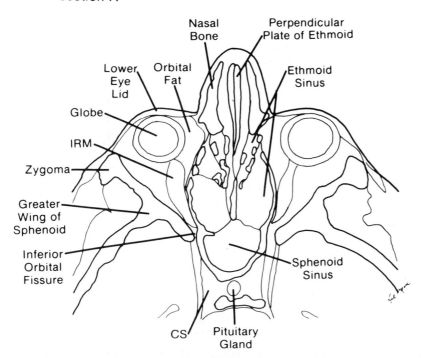

Figure 6.1. A and **B:** Section A, at the level of the inferior orbital fissure. The inferior rectus muscle *(IRM)* is seen. It provides the action of adduction and rotation of the globe downward and inward. Note that, in addition to being at the level of the inferior orbital fissure, a majority of the ethmoid and sphenoid sinuses are seen. These landmarks are helpful in recognizing the inferior rectus muscle. The cavernous sinus *(CS)* is seen owing to the use of intravenous contrast medium. The greater wing of the sphenoid and zygomatic bones form the lateral wall of the orbit.

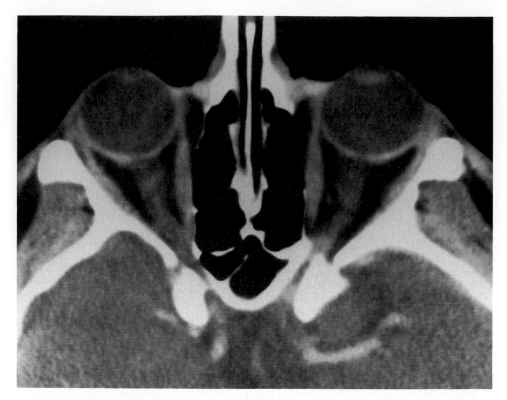

Section B

Figure 6.2. A and **B:** Section B, through the optic nerve. The optic nerve, which varies in length from 3 to 5 cm, is seen coursing posteriorly from its insertion into the sclera to the optic canal. The medial rectus muscle *(MRM)* is adjacent to the ethmoid sinus. It has the largest diameter of the six ocular muscles. The action that the medial rectus performs is adduction of the globe. The lateral rectus muscle *(LRM),* which is adjacent to the lateral wall, abducts the globe. Lateral to the optic canal is the superior orbital fissure. On axial scans it often is difficult to distinguish the superior orbital fissure from the optic canal. The only separation between these two foramen is the optic strut.

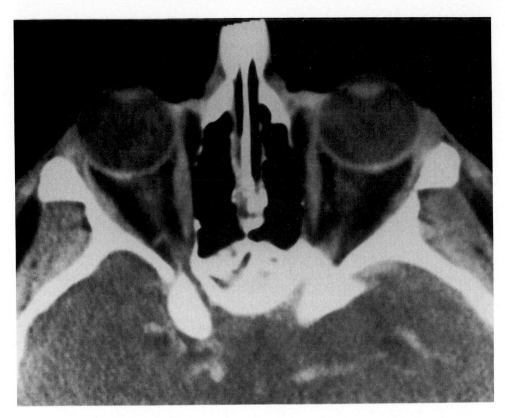

A

Section C

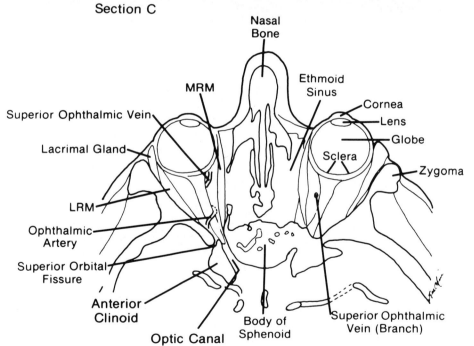

B

Figure 6.3. A and **B:** Section C, 3 mm cephalad to the previous scan. The ophthalmic artery is crossing over the optic nerve. There is good visualization of the lens bilaterally. *LRM,* lateral rectus muscle; *MRM,* medial rectus muscle.

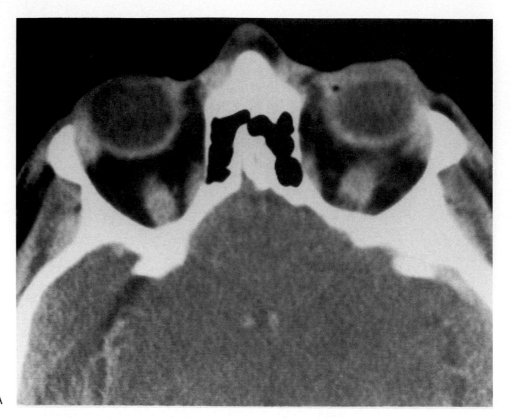

A

Section D

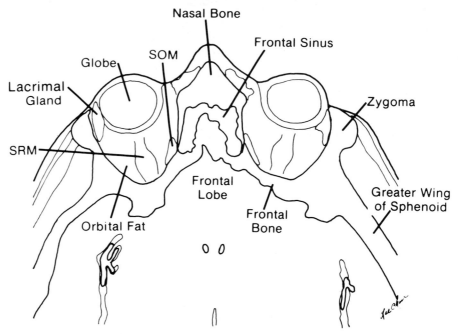

B

Figure 6.4. A and **B:** Section D, through the superior orbital cavity. The superior rectus muscle *(SRM)* is the longest of the ocular muscles. Its action is adduction, upward, and medial rotation of the eyeball. Note that there is now visualization of the frontal lobe of the brain, and few sinusal structures are seen when compared to the previous slices. Recognizing these findings helps identify the superior rectus muscle. The superior oblique muscle *(SOM)* is seen in the medial aspect of the orbit. Its action is abduction and rotation of the globe downward and outward. The tear-secreting lacrimal gland is in the lateral aspect of the orbit.

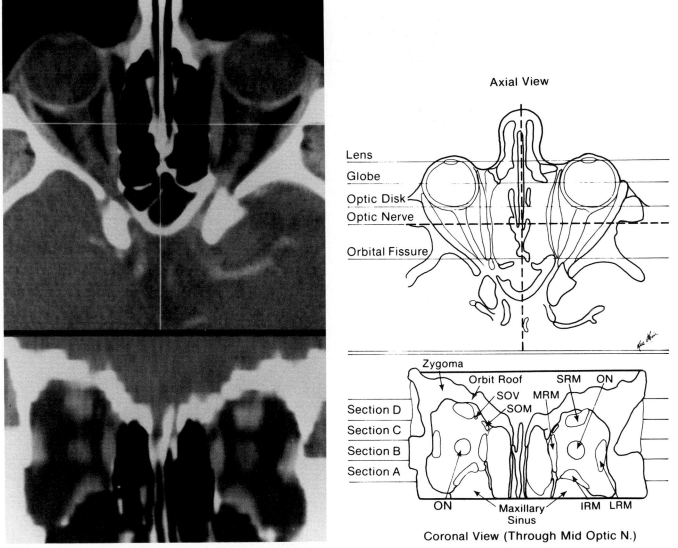

Figure 6.5. A and **B:** *(Top)* This view shows recommended areas for performing routine coronal reformations for standard axial examinations. *(Bottom)* Coronal reconstruction through the mid-optic nerve. This reconstruction demonstrates the levels at which sections A, B, C, and D (Figs. 6.1 through 6.4) were taken and their relationship to the orbital anatomy. *IRM,* inferior rectus muscle; *LRM,* lateral rectus muscle; *MRM,* medial rectus muscle; *ON,* optic nerve; *SOM,* superior oblique muscle; *SOV,* superior ophthalmic vein; *SRM,* superior rectus muscle.

References and Suggested Readings

1. Cobb SR, Yeakley JW, Lee KF, Mehinger M, Grinnell VS. Computed tomographic evaluation of ocular trauma. *Comput Radiol* 1985;9:1–9.
2. Daniels DL, Haughton VM, Williams AL, et al. Computed tomography of the optic chiasm. *Radiology* 1980;137:123–127.
3. Forbes GS. Computed tomography of the orbit. *Radiol Clin North Am* 1982;20:37–39.
4. Forbes GS, Earnest F, Waller RR. Computed tomography of orbital tumors, including late-generation scanning techniques. *Radiology* 1982;142:387–394.
5. Hammerschlag SB, Hesselink JR, Weber AL. *Computed tomography of the eye and orbit*. Norwalk, CT: Appleton-Century-Crofts, 1983.
6. Hesselink JR, Davis KR, Weber AL, et al. Radiological evaluation of orbital metastases with emphasis on computed tomography. *Radiology* 1980;137:363–366.
7. Nugent RA, Rootman J, Robertson WD, et al. Acute orbital pseudotumors: classification and CT features. *Am J Neuroradiol* 1981;2:431–436.
8. Rothfus WE, Curtin HD. Extraocular muscle enlargement: A CT review. *Radiology* 1984;151:677–681.
9. Tubman DE: Use of contrast infusion in cranial extracerebral computed tomography. *J Can Assoc Radiol* 1980;31:181–184.
10. Unger JM. Orbital apex fractures: the contribution of computed tomography. *Radiology* 1984;150:713–717.
11. Wilms G, Smits J, Baert AL. CT of the orbit: current status with high resolution computed tomography. *Neuroradiology* 1983;24:183–192.
12. Zilkha A. Multiplanar reconstruction in computed tomography of the orbit. *Comput Radiol* 1982;6:57–62.

7

Temporal Bone and Paranasal Sinuses

Temporal Bone

Characteristics such as thin sections (1–2 mm) and high spatial resolution to demonstrate intricate temporal bone anatomy have made computed tomography extremely effective in evaluating the temporal bone. High-resolution computed tomography is universally used in evaluating the temporal bone for traumatic injury and middle ear diseases such as cholesteatoma and chronic otitis media.

In the 1970s, pluridirectional tomography was considered the best method for these studies. Great advantages, such as the capability of viewing brain and bone together or showing both bone erosion and tumor when a temporal bone tumor was suspected, have made CT a superior imaging technique. CT has also eliminated the problem in pluridirectional tomography of ghost shadows simulating chronic diseases and soft tissue masses within the middle ear cavity (17).

The axial position is ordinarily used for CT of the temporal bone since it is the easiest for the patient, and most structures are demonstrated well. Scans are oriented to a plane that runs parallel to the orbitomeatal line. Coronal projections may be incorporated as an additional projection in these examinations.

Slice thickness of 2 mm or less provides optimal detail of temporal anatomy since nearly all structures are 1–2 mm in size.

Because of high inherent contrast in the temporal bone produced by the bone and air, high mAs techniques are usually not needed as would be the case if the same slice thickness were used for soft tissue scanning of the brain (25,27).

Air Cisternography

Air cisternography is an examination utilizing air as a contrast material to examine the inner ear. It is normally used for patients with hearing loss produced by small tumors of the inner ear, such as an acoustic neuroma, the most common tumor of the inner ear. Air is used because it is nontoxic, is reabsorbed and does not cause problems with future radiologic examinations, which makes it the best and safest contrast in these examinations (1,2).

With the affected ear up, the patient is tilted at an angle of about 45° by resting himself or herself on his or her lower elbow. With the head positioned so that the sagittal plane is parallel to the floor, 3–5 ml of air is injected into the subarachnoid space by lumbar puncture. The patient is left in this position for 2–4 minutes to allow the air to rise to the cerebello-pontine angle (CPA) cistern. During this period, the midsagittal plane is angled down slightly to direct the air to the CPA cistern of interest. A sensation of pressure behind the affected ear indicates that the air is probably in the correct spot. The patient is then placed in the decubitus position to keep the air in the cistern that is being examined. The head is placed so that the sagittal plane is in a lateral position. Scanning is done at a couch index and slice thickness of 1–2 mm through the internal auditory canal.

Magnetic resonance imaging (MRI) has become the standard method for evaluating the inner ear for acoustic neuromas. Air cisternography is reserved for patients who cannot undergo or tolerate MRI.

Paranasal Sinuses

CT has become increasingly important to the diagnosis of inflammatory diseases and malignant lesions of the paranasal sinuses. Its capability of demonstrating traumatic or pathologic bone destruction and of outlining soft tissue changes simultaneously have made planning of radiation therapy and surgery much easier (13,18,21,22).

The most important contribution CT has made in sinus imaging is showing lesion extension into surrounding structures.

Positioning

For routine examinations the patient's head is placed in the axial position with the infraorbitomeatal line perpendicular to the room floor. A lateral localizer is employed and scanning is done in a plane parallel to the infraorbitomeatal line. The first slice starts at the hard palate and scanning continues through the frontal sinus.

Although the axial position is adequate as a baseline study in a majority of paranasal examinations, there will be instances when scanning may also need to be performed in the coronal position (see Prone and Supine Coronal Positioning, Chapter 5 [Sella]). The coronal position is helpful in defining intracranial extension of sinus, nasopharyngeal, and nasal tumors. In the coronal position, scanning is done in a plane perpendicular to the infraorbitomeatal line if possible. If it appears that the patient cannot maintain the coronal position, then coronal reformations will suffice.

Technique

In paranasal sinus examinations a 3–6-mm slice thickness and couch index are generally used. When doing examinations where there is a question of bone destruction, bone windows should always be taken so there is demonstration of bone detail.

CONTRAST ENHANCEMENT

The use of intravenous contrast material is recommended for routine scanning. Its use can be helpful in defining intracranial tumor extension and outlining neoplastic margins (13,18,24). A bolus/drip infusion technique will generally give good diagnostic results.

Screening of the Sinuses for Inflammatory Disease

This technique, which has been described by Babbel et al. is recommended as a presurgical screening for patients prior to endoscopic sinonasal surgery (4). Endoscopic sinonasal surgery is a procedure that is used in the evaluation and treatment of sinonasal inflammatory disease that does not respond to the proper medical therapy (16,23).

One of the goals of this screening examination is to identify nonreversible disease, that is, the component of the disease that has not responded to conservative medical therapy. Therefore, a key to producing a diagnostic examination is to eliminate as much reversible disease as possible. The manner in which this can be done is through a course of antibiotics administered before scanning. Use of sympathomimetic nasal spray given 15 minutes before the exam, followed by vigorous nose blowing, thereby eliminates reversible disease.

For this screening procedure, the patient is placed in the prone coronal position with the head hyperextended, resting on chin. This position keeps free fluid out of the infundibulum. If the patient is unable to tolerate the prone position then the supine position is utilized. The gantry angle is perpendicular to the hard palate to obtain direct coronal images. A 5-mm slice thickness and couch index are used from the posterior margin of the sphenoid sinus to the anterior margin of the posterior ethmoid. From the anterior margin of the posterior ethmoid to the anterior margin of the frontal sinus a 3-mm slice thickness and couch index are used.

For this particular examination, intravenous contrast is not used.

Normal Anatomy of the Temporal Bone

The following images (Figs. 7.1 through 7.4) of the left temporal bone were obtained in the axial position at 65 mA, exposure time of 7.7 sec, 360° scan angle, and a 2-mm slice thickness and couch index. The images were magnified to a 6-cm field size through a software program known either as targeting or on-line reconstruction.

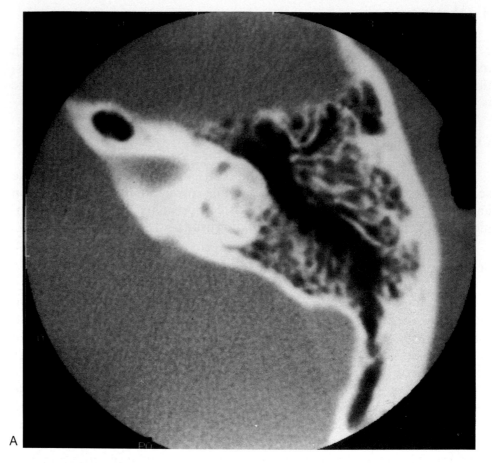

A

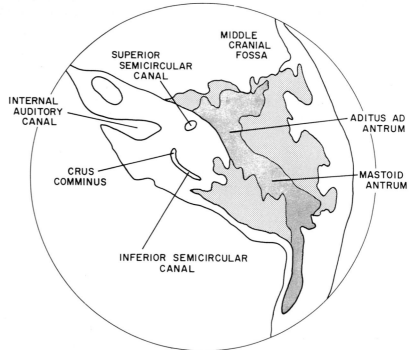

B

Figure 7.1. A and **B** were taken 4 mm below the orbitomeatal line.

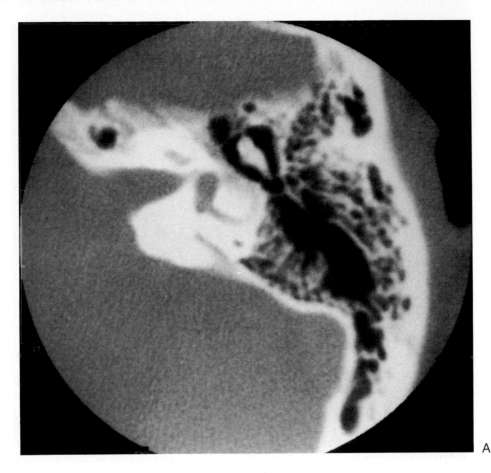

A

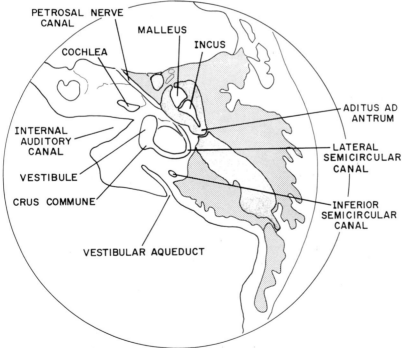

B

Figure 7.2. A and **B** were taken 6 mm caudal to the orbitomeatal line.

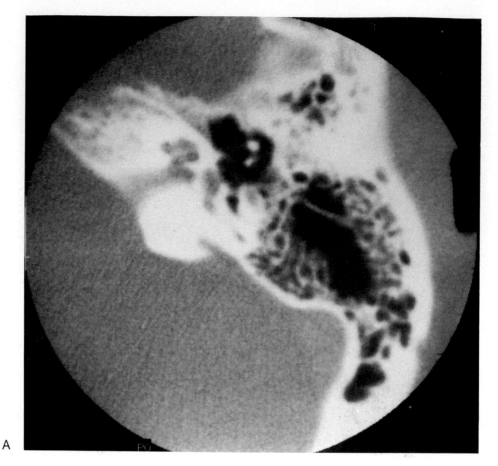

A

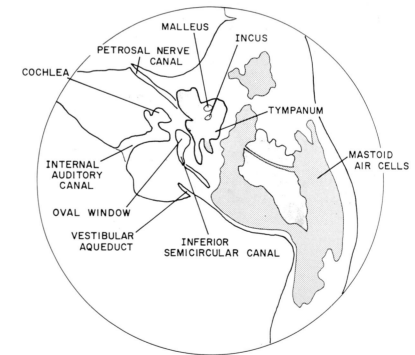

B

Figure 7.3. A and **B** were taken 8 mm caudal to orbitomeatal line.

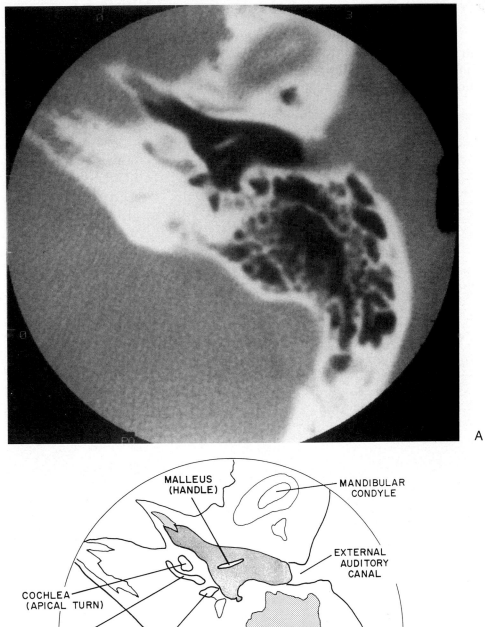

A

B

Figure 7.4. A and **B** were taken 10 mm caudal to orbitomeatal line.

Normal Anatomy of the Paranasal Sinuses

The following series of sinus images (Figs. 7.5 through 7.8) were obtained in the axial position at 65 mA, exposure time of 6.2 sec, and a 360° scan angle. The slice thickness and couch index were 5 mm. For further information on the entire sinuses, refer to Chapters 4 and 6.

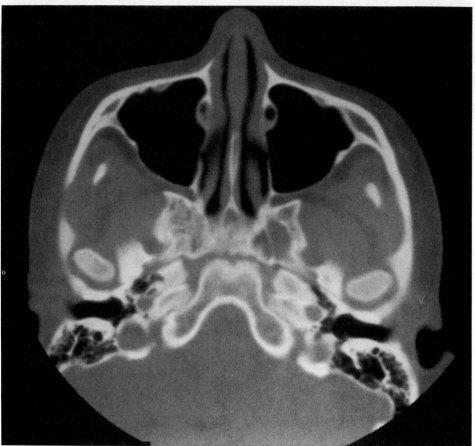

A

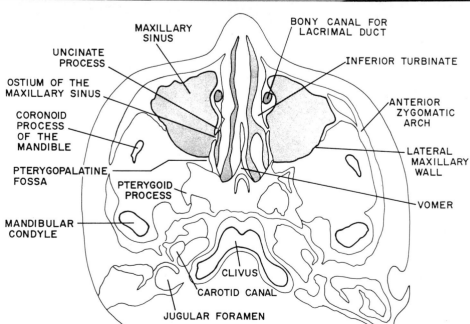

B

Figure 7.5. A and **B** were taken 2 cm above the hard palate.

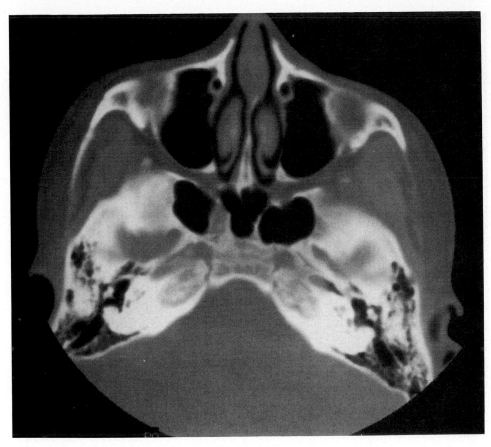

A

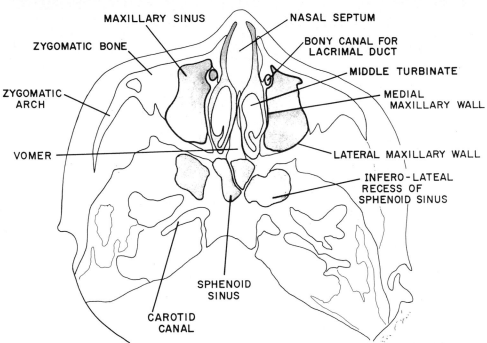

B

Figure 7.6. A and **B** were taken 5 mm cephalad to the previous slice.

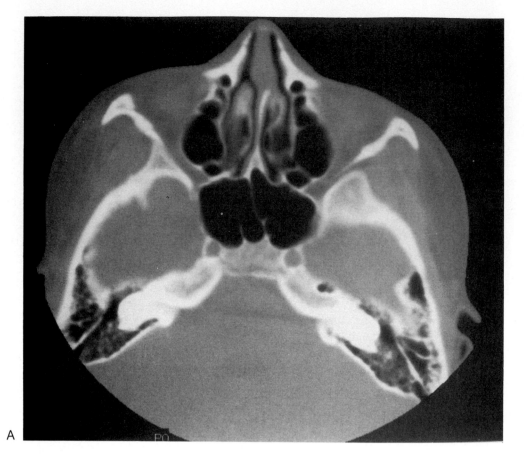

A

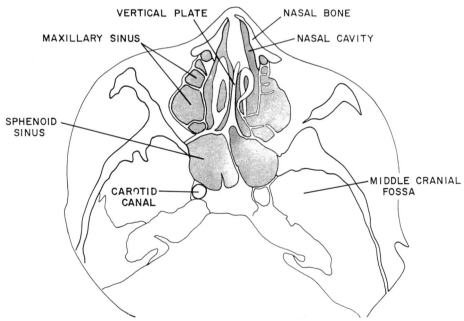

B

Figure 7.7. A and **B** were taken 5 mm cephalad to the previous slice.

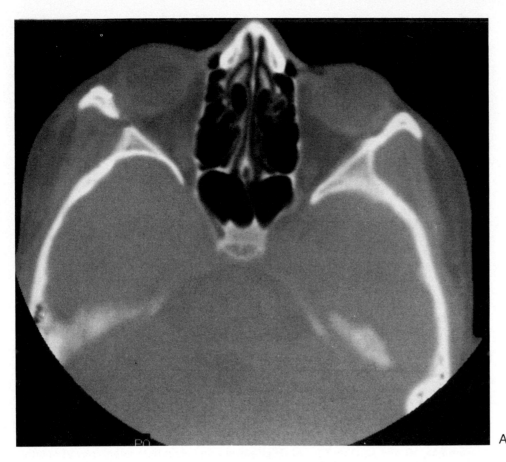

A

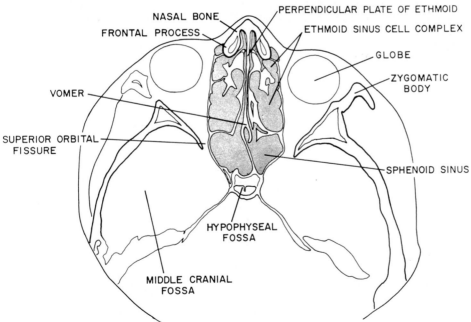

B

Figure 7.8. A and **B** were taken 5 mm cephalad to the previous slice.

References and Suggested Readings

1. Anderson R, Diehl J, Maravilla K, et al. Computerized axial tomography with air contrast of the cerebellopontine angle and internal auditory canal. *Laryngoscope* 1981; 91:1083–1096.
2. Anderson R, Olson J, Dorwart R, et al. CT air-contrast scanning of the internal auditory canal. *Ann Otol Rhinol Laryngol* 1982;91:501–505.
3. Aviahami E, Horowitz I, Cohn DF. Computed tomography of the temporo-mandibular joint. *Comput Radiol* 1984;8:211–216.
4. Babbel R, Harnsberger HR, Nelson B, et al. Optimization of techniques in screening CT of the sinuses. *Am J Roetgenol* 1991;157:1093–1098.
5. Betz BW, Wiener MD. Air in the temporomandibular joint fossa: CT sign of temporal bone fracture. *Radiology* 1991;180:463–466.
6. Bilaniuk LT, Zimmerman RA. Computed tomography in evaluation of the paranasal sinuses. *Radiol Clin North Am* 1982;20:51–66.
7. Chakeres DW, Kapila A, La Masters D. Soft-tissue abnormalities of the external auditory canal: Subject review of CT findings. *Radiology* 1985;156:105–109.
8. Chakeres DW, Spiegel PK. A systematic technique for comprehensive evaluation of the temporal bone by computed tomography. *Radiology* 1983;146:97–106.
9. Chakeres DW, Weider DJ. Computed tomography of the ossicles. *Neuroradiology* 1985;27:99–107.
10. Dodd GD, Jing BS. *Diagnostic radiology of the paranasal sinuses.* 2nd ed. Baltimore, Williams and Wilkins, (in press).
11. Dolan KD, Jacoby CG, Smoker WRK. The radiology of facial fractures. *Radiol Clin North Am* 1984;4:577–663.
12. Fritz P, Rieden K, Lenarz T, et al. Radiological evaluation of temporal bone disease: high-resolution computed tomography versus conventional x-ray diagnosis. *Br J Radiol* 1989;62:107–113.
13. Hasso AN. CT of tumors and tumor-like conditions of the paranasal sinuses. *Radiol Clin North Am* 1984;22:119–130.
14. Holland BA, Brant-Zawadski M. High resolution CT of temporal bone trauma. *Am J Roetgenol* 1984;143:391–395.
15. Isono M, Murata K, Ohta F, et al. High-resolution computed tomography of auditory ossicles. *Acta Radiol* 1990;31:27–31.
16. Kennedy DW, Zinreich SJ, Rosenbaum AE, et al. Functional endoscopic sinus surgery: theory and diagnostic evaluation. *Arch Otolaryngol Head Neck Surg* 1985;111:576–582.
17. Lufkin R, Barni JJ, Glen W, et al. Comparison of computed tomography and pluridirectional tomography of the temporal bone. *Radiology* 1982;143:715–718.
18. Mancuso AA, Hanafee WN. *Computed tomography of the head and neck.* Baltimore, Williams & Wilkins, 1982.
19. Marmolya G, Wiesen EJ, Yagan R, et al. Paranasal sinuses: low dose CT. *Radiology* 1991;181:689–691.
20. Mafee MF, Chow JM, Meyers R. Functional endoscopic sinus surgery: anatomy, CT screening, indications and complications. *Am J Roetgenol* 1993;160:735–744.
21. Nakagawa H, Wolf BS. Delineation of lesions of the base of skull by computed tomography. *Radiology* 1977;124:75–80.
22. Parsons C, Hodson N. Computed tomography of paranasal sinus tumors. *Radiology* 1979;132:641–645.
23. Rice DH. Basic surgical techniques and variations of endoscopic sinus surgery. *Otolaryngol Clin North Am* 1989;22:713–726.
24. Schatz CJ, Becker TS. Normal CT anatomy of the paranasal sinuses. *Radiol Clin North Am* 1984;22:107–118.
25. Shaffer K. Computed tomography of the temporal bone. *Radiographics* 1981;1:62–63.
26. Som PM. CT of the paranasal sinuses. *Neuroradiology* 1985;27:189–201.
27. Taylor S. CT of the petrous bone. In: *Computed tomography of the whole body.* Vol. 2. St. Louis: C.V. Mosby, 1983;1009–1016.
28. Thawley SE, Gado M, Fuller TR. Computerized tomography in the evaluation of head and neck lesions. *Laryngoscope* 1978;88:451–459.
29. Torizuka T, Hayakawa K, Satoh Y, et al. High-resolution CT of the temporal bone: a modified baseline. *Radiology* 1992;184:109–111.
30. Virapongse C, Rothman SLG, Sasaki C, Kier EL. The role of high resolution computed tomography in evaluation disease of the middle ear. *J Comput Assist Tomogr* 1982;6:711–720.
31. Weber AL, Tadmor R, Davis R, et al. Malignant tumors of the sinuses: radiologic evaluation, including CT scanning with clinical and pathologic correlation. *Neuroradiology* 1978;16:433–448.
32. Zonneveld FW, Van Waes PFGM, Damsma H, et al. Direct multiplanar computed tomography of the petrous bone. *Radiographics* 1983;3:400–422.

Neck

Positioning

The patient is placed in the supine position with the neck slightly hyperextended, shoulders relaxed, and arms to the sides. A lateral localizer is obtained for positioning. For scans of the entire neck, scanning starts at the occiput and continues to T_1.

Technique

Generally, a 5–10-mm slice thickness and couch index are used for routine examinations of the neck. If detailed examinations and fine reformations are needed, 5-mm or smaller sections are suggested.

Several artifacts can degrade image quality when scanning the neck. Breathing, swallowing, and dental fillings can hinder an examination.

Motion artifact caused by breathing and swallowing can significantly reduce image clarity around parts of the airway. When performing neck examinations, the patient should hold his or her breath, and the shortest scan time possible should be used. To prevent motion artifact produced by swallowing, the patient is asked to bite gently with the lips on the partially extended tip of the tongue (6).

Dental artifacts can be reduced by tilting the gantry, or the patient can be asked to open and close his or her mouth. If the latter technique is used, it is important that the patient be instructed to limit movement to the mandible. Often dental artifacts can be avoided by simply asking the patient to remove his or her dentures before the examination.

Beam-hardening artifact at the level of the shoulders is a normal problem with neck examinations, particularly in obese or very muscular patients. Increasing the milliamperage and using the swimmer's view can help to reduce beam-hardening artifact.

CONTRAST ENHANCEMENT

Intravenous (IV) contrast can be important in the assessment of soft tissue masses and their extension. IV contrast also makes it easier to visualize vascular structures. A 30-ml bolus of contrast medium followed by a 150-ml rapid drip infusion gives the maintained plasma iodine levels needed for neck examinations. In examinations where vascular structures must be accurately defined from lymph nodes or masses, rapid scanning with use of a power injector should be considered. An injection rate of 0.5–1 ml/sec is suggested (2). For clinical considerations in the use of power injectors, dynamic scanning and other contrast enhancements, see Contrast Enhancement (Chapter 9).

Normal Anatomy of the Neck

The following series of neck images (Figs. 8.1 through 8.12) were obtained at 65 mA, exposure time of 5 sec, and 360° scan angle. The slice thickness and couch index were 6 mm. For intravenous contrast enhancement, a bolus/drip method was used.

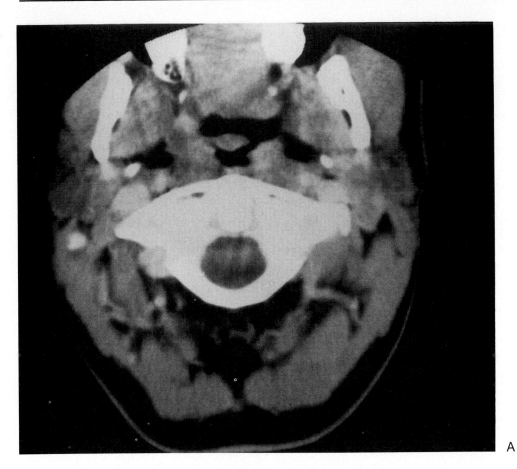

A

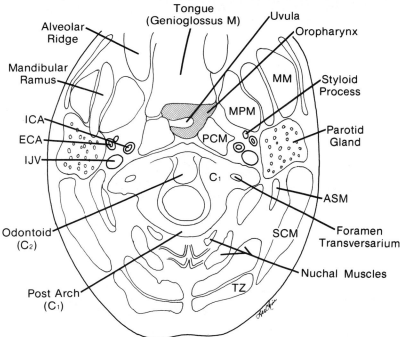

B

Figure 8.1 A and **B:** CT scan taken at C_1. *ASM*, anterior scalene muscle; *ECA*, external carotid artery; *ICA*, internal carotid artery; *IJV*, internal jugular vein; *MM*, masseter muscle; *MPM*, medial pterygoid muscle; *PCM*, pharyngeal constrictor muscle; *SCM*, sternocleidomastoid muscle; *TZ*, trapezius muscle.

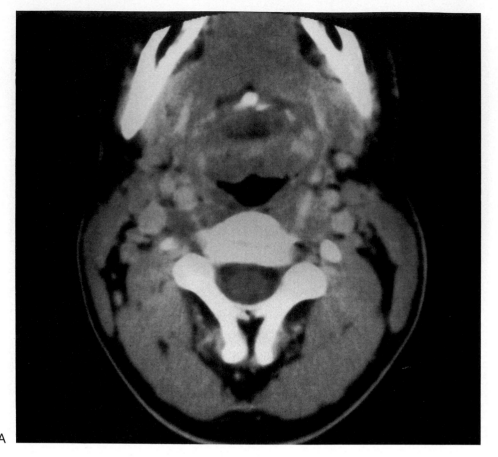

A

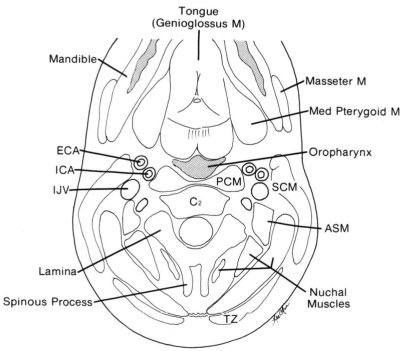

B

Figure 8.2. A and **B:** CT scan through C₂. *ASM,* anterior scalene muscle; *ECA,* external carotid artery; *ICA,* internal carotid artery; *IJV,* internal jugular vein; *PCM,* pharyngeal constrictor muscle; *SCM,* sternocleidomastoid muscle; *TZ,* trapezius muscle.

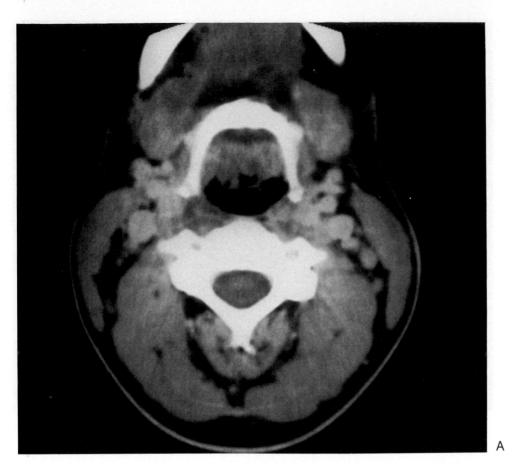

A

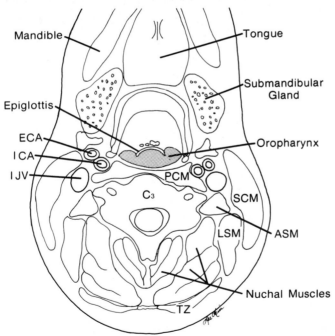

B

Figure 8.3. A and **B:** Cross-section at C₃. Note the thyroid bone, which has a horseshoe-shaped appearance. There is some saliva trapped in the right epiglottis region in this slice performed in suspended respiration. *ASM,* anterior scalene muscle; *ECA,* external carotid artery; *ICA,* internal carotid artery; *IJV,* internal jugular vein; *LSM,* levator scapular muscle; *PCM,* pharyngeal constrictor muscle; *SCM,* sternocleidomastoid muscle; *TZ,* trapezius muscle.

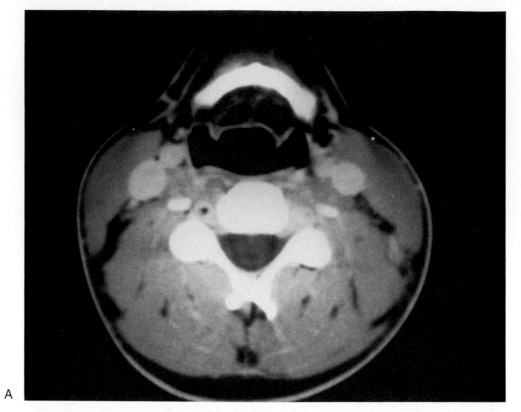

A

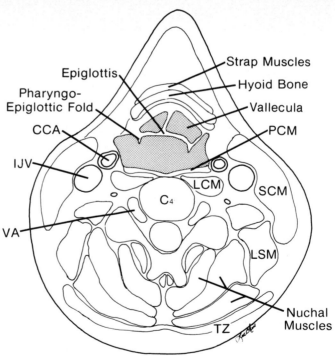

B

Figure 8.4. A and **B:** CT scan at the top of C$_4$. *CCA,* common carotid artery. *IJV,* internal jugular vein; *LCM,* longus colli muscle; *LSM,* levator scapular muscle; *PCM,* pharyngeal constrictor muscle; *SCM,* sternocleidomastoid muscle; *TZ,* trapezius muscle; *VA,* vertebral artery.

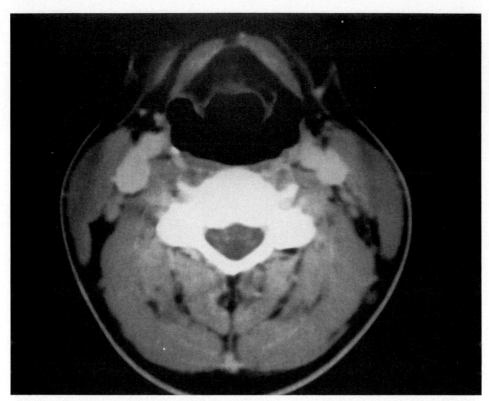

A

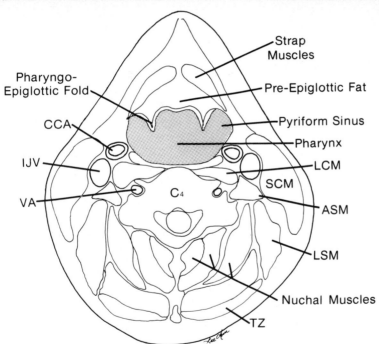

B

Figure 8.5. A and **B:** Cross-section at the middle of C$_4$. There is excellent distention of the pyriform sinus owing to the use of the valsalva maneuver. *ASM*, anterior scalene muscle; *CCA*, common carotid artery; *IJV*, internal jugular vein; *LCM*, longus colli muscle; *LSM*, levator scapular muscle; *SCM*, sternocleidomastoid muscle; *TZ*, trapezius muscle; *VA*, vertebral artery.

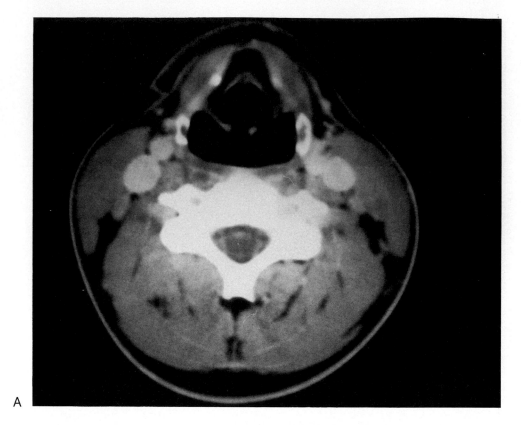

A

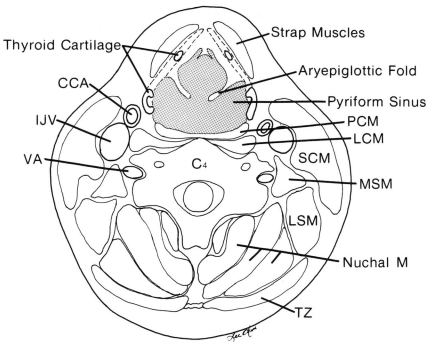

B

Figure 8.6. **A** and **B:** Cross-section at the bottom of C₄, which is 3 mm caudad to the previous section. The thyroid cartilage is beginning to be visualized. The aryepiglottic fold is seen separating the pyriform sinus and laryngeal vestibule. *CCA*, common carotid artery; *IJV*, internal jugular vein; *LCM*, longus colli muscle; *LSM*, levator scapular muscle; *MSM*, middle scalene muscle; *PCM*, pharyngeal constrictor muscle; *SCM*, sternocleidomastoid muscle; *TZ*, trapezius muscle; *VA*, vertebral artery.

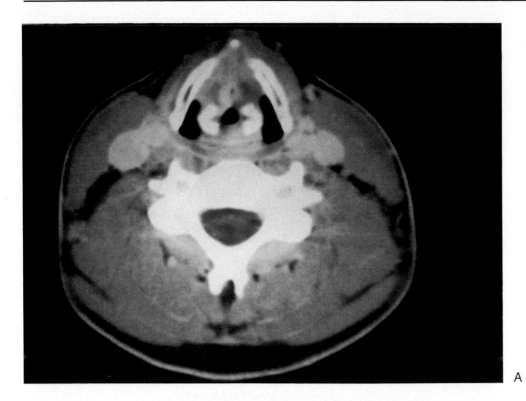

A

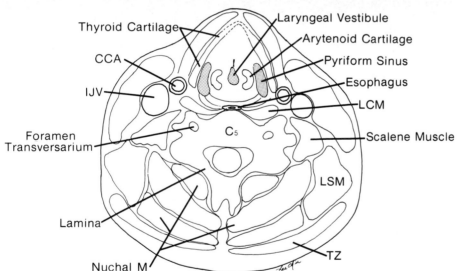

B

Figure 8.7. A and **B:** CT scan at C₅. The thyroid and arytenoid cartilage are well visualized. *CCA,* common carotid artery; *IJV,* internal jugular vein; *LCM,* longus colli muscle; *LSM,* levator scapular muscle; *TZ,* trapezius muscle.

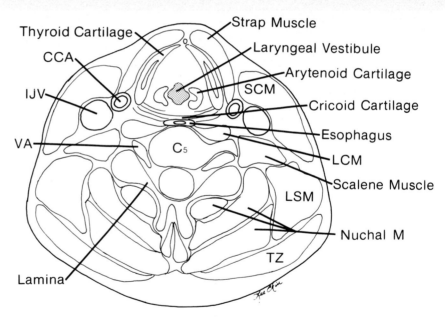

Figure 8.8. A and **B:** Cross-section 3 mm caudad to the previous slice shows that the pyriform sinus is no longer demonstrated. *CCA,* common carotid artery; IJV, internal jugular vein; *LCM,* longus colli muscle; *LSM,* levator scapular muscle; *SCM,* sternocleidomastoid muscle; *TZ,* trapezius muscle; *VA,* vertebral artery.

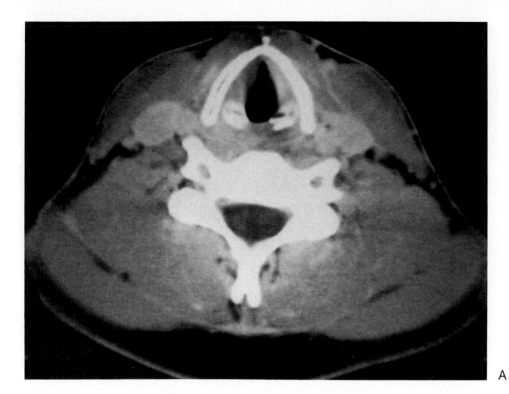

A

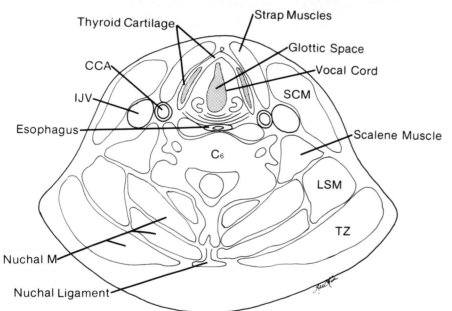

B

Figure 8.9. A and **B:** Cross-section at the top of C_6. The vocal cords can be identied at this level. *CCA*, common carotid artery; *IJV*, internal jugular vein; *LSM*, levator scapular muscle; *SCM*, sternocleidomastoid muscle; *TZ*, trapezius muscle.

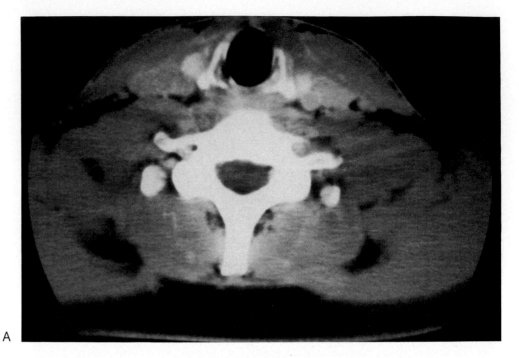

Figure 8.10. A and **B:** CT scan at the bottom of C₆. The cricoid cartilage is beginning to be seen. There is partial visualization of the thyroid gland. *CCA,* common carotid artery; *IJV,* internal jugular vein; *LCM,* longus colli muscle; *LSM,* levator scapular muscle; *SCM,* sternocleidomastoid muscle; *TZ,* trapezius muscle; *VA,* vertebral artery.

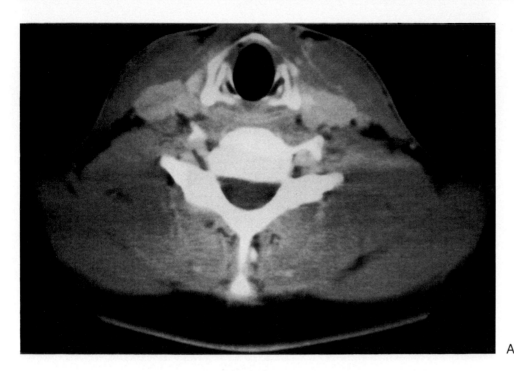

A

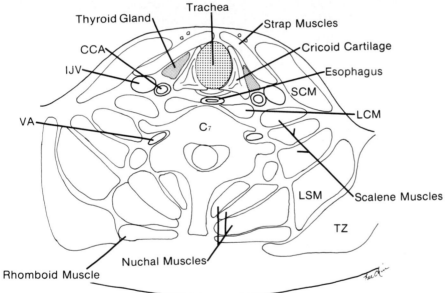

B

Figure 8.11. A and **B:** Cross-section at the top of C₇. *CCA,* common carotid artery; *IJV,* internal jugular vein; *LCM,* longus colli muscle; *LSM,* levator scapular muscle; *SCM,* sternocleidomastoid muscle; *TZ,* trapezius muscle; *VA,* vertebral artery.

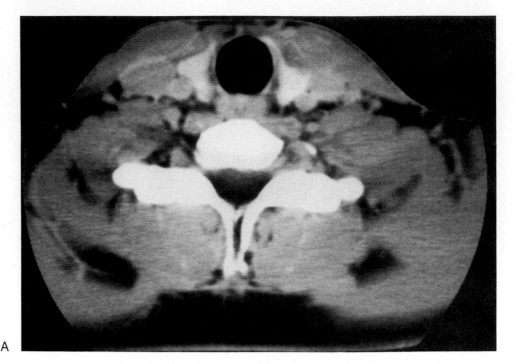

A

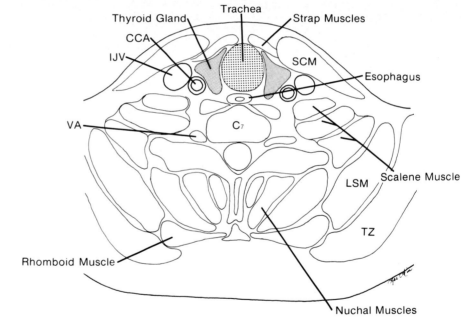

B

Figure 8.12. A and **B:** CT scan through the bottom of C$_7$. Generally, the thyroid gland is easily identified because of its high attenuation value, which results from the iodine content within the thyroid gland. After contrast administration, the thyroid gland becomes much denser. *CCA,* common carotid artery; *IJV,* internal jugular vein; *LSM,* levator scapular muscle; *SCM,* sternocleidomastoid muscle; *TZ,* trapezius muscle; *VA,* vertebral artery.

References and Suggested Readings

1. Carter BL. Computed tomographic scanning in head and neck tumors. *Otolaryngol Clin North Am* 1980;13:449–457.
2. Gay SB, Pevarski DR, Phillips CD, et al. Dynamic CT of the neck. *Radiology* 1991; 180:284–285.
3. Ginsberg LE. Neoplastic diseases affecting the central skull base: CT and MR imaging. *Am J Roetgenol* 1992;159:581–589.
4. Harnsbergger HR, Osborn AG. Differential diagnosis of head and neck lesions based on their space of origin. *Am J Roetgenol* 1991;157:147–159.
5. Mancuso AA, Hanafee WN. *Computed tomography of the head and neck*. Baltimore: Williams & Wilkins, 1982.
6. Martinez CR, Gayler BW, Kashima H, et al. Computed tomography of the neck. *Radiographics* 1983;3:9–25.
7. Michael AS, Mafee MF, Valvassori GE, et al. Dynamic computed tomography of the head and neck: differential diagnostic value. *Radiology* 1985;154:413–419.
8. Miller MB, Rao VM, Tom BL. Cystic masses of the head and neck: pitfalls in CT and MR interpretation. *Am J Roetgenol* 1992;159:601–607.
9. Rauschkolb EN, Keen SJ, Patel S. High dose computed tomography in the evaluation of low attenuation lesions in the neck. *J Comput Tomogr* 1983;7:159–166.
10. Reede DL, Whelan MA, Bergeron RT. CT of the soft tissue structures of the neck. *Radiol Clin North Am* 1984;22:239–250.
11. Russell EJ, D'Angelo CM, Zimmerman RD, et al. Cervical disk herniation: CT demonstration after contrast enhancement. *Radiology* 1984;152:703–712.
12. Thawley SE, Gado M, Fuller TR. Computerized tomography in the evaluation of head and neck lesions. *Laryngoscope* 1978;88:451–459.
13. Vibhakar SD, Eckhauser C, Bellon EM. Computed tomography of the nasopharynx and neck. *J Comput Tomogr* 1983;7:259–265.

Chest

Positioning

Generally, scans of the chest are done with the patient supine, arms elevated above the head. A posterior–anterior (PA) localizer (Fig. 9.1) is taken, with the first slice starting at the apices. The examination continues through the adrenal glands. Scanning through the adrenal glands is done to evaluate for adrenal metastasis.

Technique

A 10-mm slice thickness and couch index are used for most examinations of the chest. Smaller sections (3–5 mm) may be needed in instances such as small-lesion localization.

Knowing the relationship of the esophagus to other mediastinal structures can be very important, particularly in cases when it can be compressed by and indistinguishable from a lesion. For opacification of the esophagus, esophageal cream containing a low percentage of barium sulfate can be very useful in defining the esophagus. The cream coats the mucosa of the esophagus without causing artifact.

RESPIRATION

To obtain optimal chest examinations, suspended respiration is mandatory to avoid motion artifact. With the introduction of third- and fourth-generation scanners, exposure times of 1–3 sec have helped eliminate the problem of respiratory and cardiac motion.

Inspiration, expiration, and mid-inspiration do not appear to affect the quality of the examination. The major consideration is that the patient hold his or her breath the same way for each slice to avoid anatomical fluctuation. Use of suspended respiration at resting volume appears to be most favorable for chest examinations, but for this to be successful it is important that the patient be given a thorough explanation of what is to be done.

POWER INJECTOR

Routine use of the power injector when indicated in computed tomography offers significant advantages and overcomes the previously stated shortcomings of drip infusions and hand bolus injections. Advantages of power injection are:

1. Accurate reproducible volumes and flows.
2. Elimination of the inherent problem of contrast media viscosity.
3. Elimination of subjecting personnel to radiation exposure by standing in the scanning room during hand injections.

When utilizing a power injector, it is suggested that a catheter size of 18–19 gauge be used. A catheter of this size allows greater flow of contrast. Whenever using a power injector, it is extremely important to first read the users' manual; some manufacturers have a minimum catheter size that is recommended for use. It is suggested that butterflies with metal needles not be used, particularly in the antecubital fossa. Chance of extravasation increase in this anatomical location. This occurs as a result of the patients raising their arm above their head; as they do this there is a tendency to bend at the elbow, increasing the likelihood of the metal needle puncturing the vein wall.

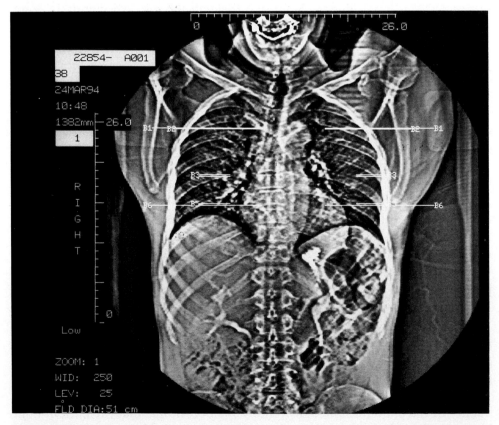

Figure 9.1. PA localizer used to determine the slice position for a chest examination. The white lines represent the location of a cross-sectional image.

CONTRAST ENHANCEMENT

Use of an intravenous (IV) contrast medium in mediastinum examinations can add valuable diagnostic information. In patients with a sufficient amount of mediastinal fat, gross mediastinal structures can be observed without contrast administration, but because most structures are vascular and do not attenuate photons it can be difficult to differentiate normal anatomy from abnormal structures. To overcome this difficulty, intra-vascular contrast media are needed. There are four methods of contrast administration: (1) drip infusion; (2) single bolus injection; (3) drip infusion followed by bolus injection; (4) multiple bolus injection. Regardless of the method, the total amount of iodine injected should never exceed 80 g.

For ideal results, IV injections start with placement of an intravenous catheter with a heparin lock to prevent clotting. As previously stated, an 18–19-gauge catheter is used so a profitable flow rate is ensured. The catheter ideally is placed at the antecubital fossa of the arm in the basilic venous system, facilitating direct flow to the superior vena cava (Fig. 9.2). Hand veins should be avoided for this purpose if possible. This is because rapid iodine flow to the heart would be completely defeated because of the long route and numerous venous valves involved.

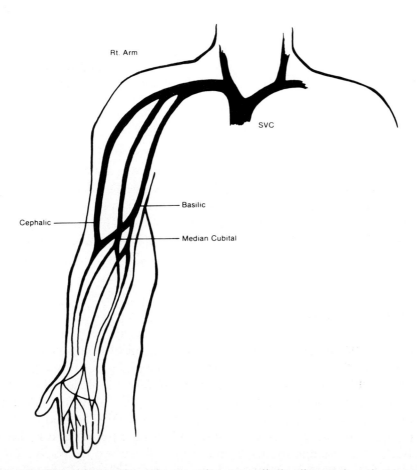

Figure 9.2. This illustration shows why a medially directed catheter placement is preferred. The route of the basilic vein to the superior vena cava (SVC) is more direct than that of the cephalic vein.

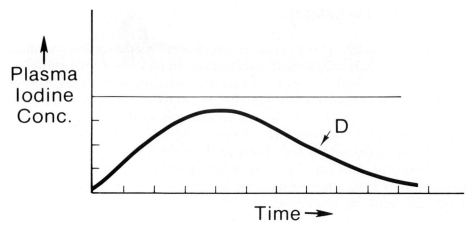

Figure 9.3. Drip infusion. The curved line *D*, which represents a drip infusion, demonstrates the slow rise in plasma iodine concentration. Note that this line never gets above the horizontal line, which represents the plasma iodine concentration needed for optimal opacification. (Modified from Burman et al. *Radiol Clin North Am* 1982;20:15–220; with permission.)

Nausea or vomiting is often induced when iodine is injected rapidly and in large volumes. To reduce the chance of vomiting, the patient should have nothing by mouth 4 hours before the examination.

Methods of Injection

DRIP INFUSION

Use of a drip infusion of contrast medium (Fig. 9.3) generally does not give ideal enhancement. Inconsistent flow rates are a major problem with the drip infusion technique. Factors such as needle size, bottle height, solution viscosity, and tubing length contribute to this inconsistency. The inconsistent flow rate causes a slow rise in the plasma iodine concentration, and generally intravascular structures stay at an isodense level of enhancement because the contrast medium is diluted and has circulated out of the intravascular space by the time scanning takes place.

SINGLE BOLUS INFUSION

A single bolus injection (Fig. 9.4) of 60–100 ml of contrast medium injected by hand or 5 ml/sec by power injector usually gives immediate intravascular opacification, which lasts approximately 30–60 sec. For optimal results, scanning should be done within 60 sec. After this time period, there is a rapid decrease in plasma iodine concentration. This method works well when a small, specific area is in question. If a longer period of opacification is desired, a slow single bolus by hand or 1–3 ml/sec by power injector may be used. For both injection methods, scanning begins 7–9 sec (average normal antecubital vein to left ventricular circulation) after the start of the bolus (Fig. 9.5A,B).

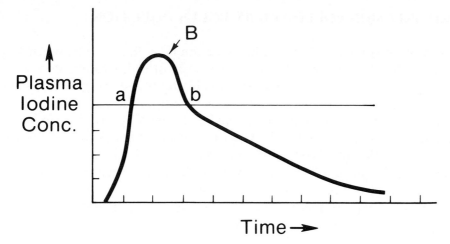

Figure 9.4. Single bolus injection. The curved line *B,* which represents a bolus, shows a rapid rise in the plasma iodine concentration. Line *a–b* represents the duration of optimal opacification (Modified from Burman et al. *Radiol Clin North Am* 1982;20:15–22, with permission.)

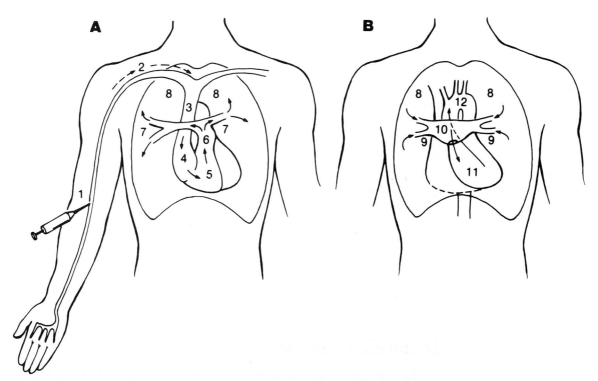

Figure 9.5. (A) Average normal circulation time for contrast to arrive in the following structures from a right antecubital vein injection. From right antecubital vein *(1)* to right subclavian vein *(2)* 0.5 sec, to superior vena cava *(3)* 1.0 sec, to right atrium *(4)* 1.5 sec, to right ventricle *(5)* 2.0 sec, to main pulmonary artery *(6)* 2.6 sec, to pulmonary arteries *(7)* 3.0 sec, to lung parenchyma *(8)* 4–5 sec. **(B)** Average normal circulation time for contrast to arrive from a right antecubital vein injection to the lung parenchyma and aortic arch. To lung parenchyma *(8)* 4–5 sec, to pulmonary veins *(9)* 6.0 sec, to left atrium *(10)* 7.0 sec, to left ventricle *(11)* 8.0 sec, to aortic arch *(12)* 9.0 sec.

DRIP INFUSION FOLLOWED BY BOLUS INJECTION

A drip infusion and then a bolus injection (Fig. 9.6) is used when a large area needs to be covered and a specific area of radiographic concern, for example, the hila or a portion of the mediastinum, needs to be highlighted.

Because of the upper low-density mediastinal fat and lack of cardiac motion, satisfactory enhancement can be obtained by a rapid drip infusion. Scanning can start immediately. Once the suspected area has been reached, a bolus injection of 40–60 ml of contrast medium is given with rapid scanning. Scanning begins 5–7 sec (average normal antecubital vein to hilar circulation) after the start of the bolus injection.

A disadvantage of this method is that it is time consuming and requires constant monitoring by a radiologist.

MULTIPLE BOLUS INJECTION

Multiple bolus contrast administration (Fig. 9.7), in which a total of 150 ml of contrast medium is administered in a bolus technique by hand or power injector, is used with dynamic scanning. This method is suggested for evaluating the entire thorax for abnormalities in the mediastinum or great vessels, including large mediastinal masses with extension or aortic aneurysms (1,2,4). This method is also of particular value for evaluating occult mediastinal tumors.

The scanning procedure begins 7–9 sec (average normal antecubital vein to left ventricular circulation) after an initial bolus injection of 30–50 ml of contrast. A continuous bolus injection of 10–15 ml by hand or, preferably, by power injector set at an injection volume of 15 ml and a flow rate of 5–7 ml/sec is made either during table indexing or during x-ray exposure. Injections are continued until the full 150 ml of contrast medium is administered. For ideal and consistent results, optimal opacification is achieved by timing the injection so that the contrast medium is at the area of interest at the time of exposure.

Advantages of this technique include a shorter examination time and maximum vessel opacification, which lead to better image quality and improved diagnostic accuracy.

If this technique is used when there is a chance that one of the brachiocephalic veins is obstructed, catheters will probably need to be placed bilaterally to ensure that the flow of contrast is not impeded. When two catheters are used, the 150 ml of contrast medium is divided equally and delivered by hand injection.

Dynamic Scanning

The object of dynamic scanning is to achieve optimal intravascular opacification throughout the mediastinum within the shortest scanning time possible so that the maximum number of slices can be obtained before the iodine concentration decreases or the study is terminated due to heat buildup. In this technique, there is no significant loss in image quality, and 16 to 20 continuous slices can be obtained in less than 4 min. This procedure works very effectively with the multiple bolus technique (Figs. 9.8, 9.9).

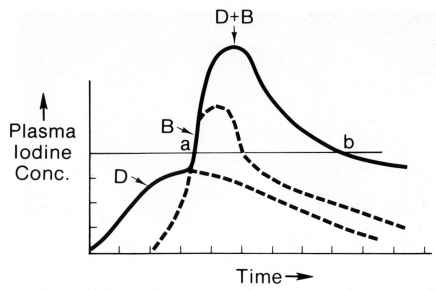

Figure 9.6. Drip infusion followed by bolus injection. The curved line *D + B* represents the summation of the drip infusion curve *(D)* and bolus injection curve *(B)*. Note that the time period of optimal opacification between *a* and *b* occurs later in the scan. (Modified from Burman et al. *Radiol Clin North Am* 1982;20:15–22; with permission.)

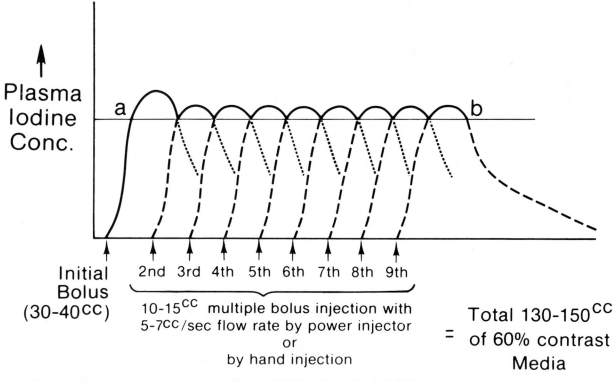

Figure 9.7. Multiple bolus injection. The time period between *A* and *B* represents the summation of the initial bolus and sequential bolus injections. Note the fairly evenly maintained plasma iodine concentration and longer duration of time. This method and rapid scanning are ideal for evaluating the entire mediastinum.

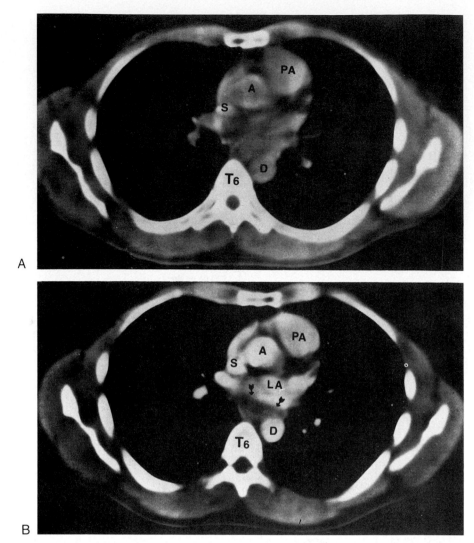

Figure 9.8. A and **B:** Unsuspected mediastinal mass. Scans **A** and **B** were obtained using exactly the same scanning parameters except that scan **A** was performed using a 40-ml bolus followed by a 110-ml drip of contrast. There is a suspected large soft tissue mass between the ascending *(A)* and descending *(D)* aortas. Because of the faint contrast enhancement, it is difficult to distinguish the left atrium from the suspected mass. Scan **B** was obtained 2 days later using the multiple-bolus technique. The nonpacified soft tissue mass *(arrows)* is now clearly seen between the left atrium *(LA)* and the T6 vertebral body. The mass proved to be bronchogenic carcinoma. *PA,* pulmonary artery; *S,* superior vena cava.

Dynamic scanning is especially useful for evaluating trauma because the examination time is short. The timing of injection is selected so the time interval between two contiguous slices is approximately 7–9 sec, which coincides with the circulation time from the antecubital vein to left ventricle. Furthermore, this timing also allows enough time for the patient to breathe and therefore helps eliminate the lingering possibility of motion artifact caused by respiration.

In order to obtain the maximum number of slices before an examination terminates because of the manufactured imposed heat units, three items

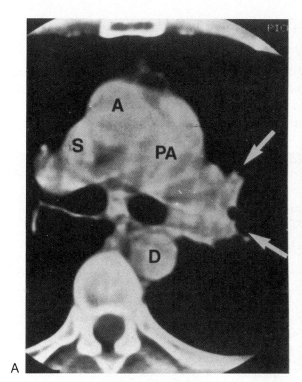 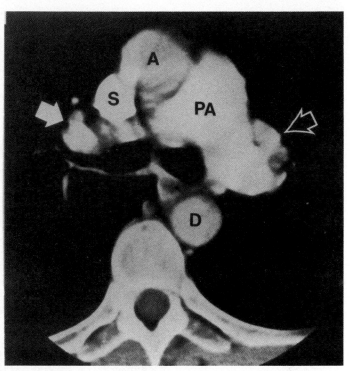

A   B

Figure 9.9. A and **B.** Pulmonary vessels. Scans **A** and **B** were obtained using exactly the same scanning parameters, except scan **A** was obtained with a rapid drip infusion. Note the irregular hilar density *(arrows)*, which initially was thought to represent a hilar mass in a patient with breast cancer. Scan **B** was obtained 1 week later using the multiple-bolus technique. Note that ''the suspected hilar mass'' has been densely opacified and can easily be recognized as the left superior pulmonary vein *(open arrow)*. The right superior pulmonary vein *(arrowhead)*, ascending aorta *(A)*, descending aorta *(D)*, pulmonary artery *(PA)*, and superior vena cava *(S)* are also well opacified.

must be considered: (1) scan rotation angle; (2) exposure time; and (3) heat units present on the tube. Use of the least amount of scan rotation and low exposure time keeps heat units down by keeping the length of time the tube is on to a minimum. This in turn allows more slices to be obtained before tube cooling is required. It is important to note that when using a low exposure time either the milliamperage or the kilovolt peak must be increased to overcome underpenetration, especially at the humeral heads. To make sure that beam hardening does not degrade image quality, a slice should be taken at the level of the humeral heads before the initial examination takes place.

Particular attention should always be paid to the heat units on the x-ray tube. To ensure that a sufficient number of slices will be accumulated before tube shutdown occurs, scanning should not start unless heat units are in the low 20% range.

This technique of scanning can be utilized by many available late-generation scanners by simply using the least amount of scan angle and shortest possible scan time. Again, it is important to increase the milliamperage to achieve better penetration. To calculate desirable milliamperage for this technique, it can be obtained using the mAs (for the individual CT chest protocol) divided by the exposure time.

High-Resolution CT (HRCT)

High-resolution CT (HRCT) is a scanning technique that optimizes spatial resolution. HRCT utilizes a high spatial-frequency reconstruction algorithm and a thin slice thickness (1–2 mm). A drawback to this technique is visualization of increased image noise. This technique has proven to be excellent for evaluating fine lung structures and airways (Fig. 9.10, A and

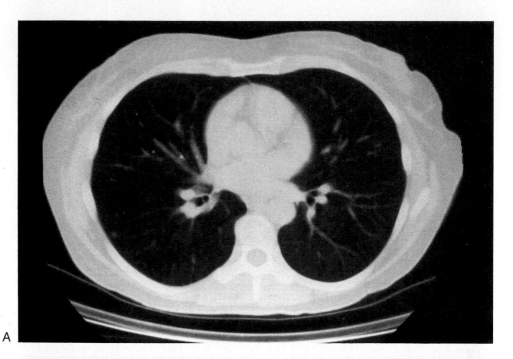

A

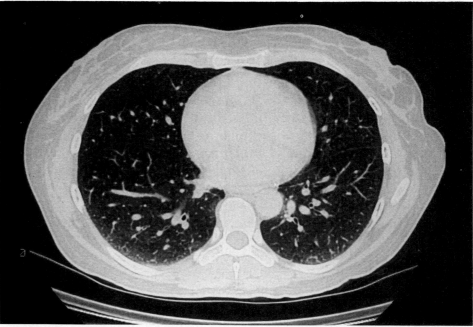

B

Figure 9.10. A and **B.** Comparison of conventional and high-resolution CT images. Image **A** taken at the level of the left atrium using a conventional technique of 130 kVp, 140 mA, 1 sec exposure, and 10-mm slice thickness. Image **B** taken at the same level as **A,** using a high-resolution technique of 130 kVp, 110 mA, 3 sec exposure, 2-mm slice thickness, and high spatial-frequency algorithm. Note the superior definition of the lung parenchyma.

B) (13,17). The area HRCT has been found particularly useful in the evaluation of patients with known diffuse lung disease such as emphysema and asbestosis.

Patients with known diffuse lung diseases are usually best evaluated with conventional CT (8–10-mm slice thickness) to evaluate the entire chests. This not only allows for evaluation of the lung parenchyma but also the mediastinum. After reviewing the initial examination and there are areas that need further assessment, then HRCT is used (Fig. 9.11, A and B). It is important to point out that there are numerous protocols for the use of HRCT, and individual departments should use what they feel comfortable with (13,16,17,25). One suggested method is to perform slices routinely at the apex, hilar area, and lung base in conjunction with conventional CT.

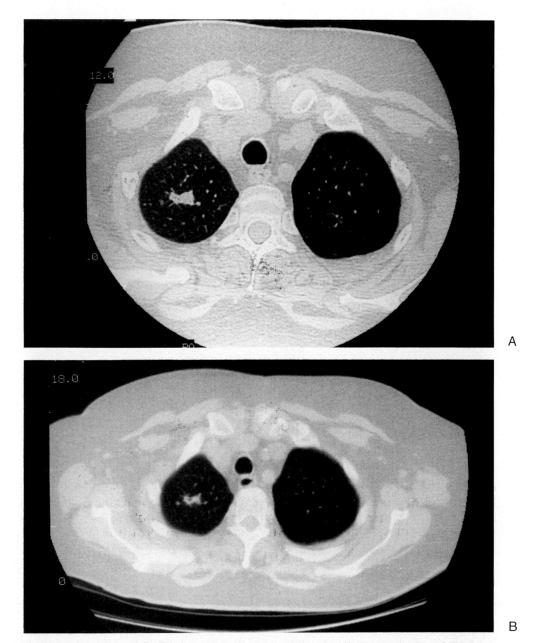

Figure 9.11. A and **B.** Right upper lung nodule. **A:** High-resolution CT image shows a well-defined right upper lobe nodule. **B:** Conventional CT image demonstrates the right upper lobe nodule with less distinction.

Mediastinal and Lung Imaging

When imaging the chest, scans at two window widths (WW) and window levels (WL) should be performed so both mediastinal and lung parenchyma can be viewed. Because these have different attenuation values, each needs to be imaged at different settings. Imaging of the mediastinum requires a narrow WW and low positive WL. Lung parenchyma requires a wide WW and a negative WL. These settings vary among CT units.

If both mediastinal and lung parenchyma are to be viewed simultaneously, most scanners have a keyboard function that offers the capability of viewing two WW's and WL's at the same time (Figs. 9.12–9.27).

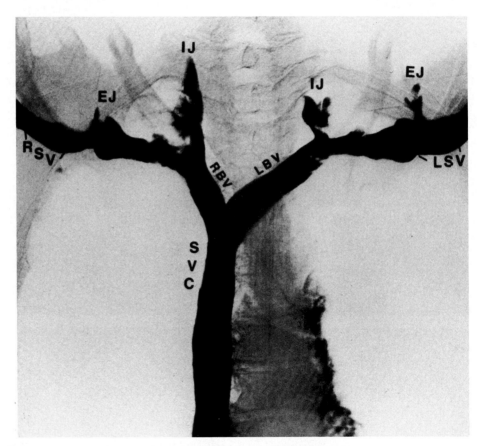

Figure 9.12. Normal venogram with bilateral injection throughout the antecubital veins. *EJ,* external jugular veins; *IJ,* internal jugular veins; *LBV,* left brachiocephalic vein; *LSV,* left subclavian vein; *RBV,* right brachiocephalic vein; *RSV,* right subclavian vein; *SVC,* superior vena cava.

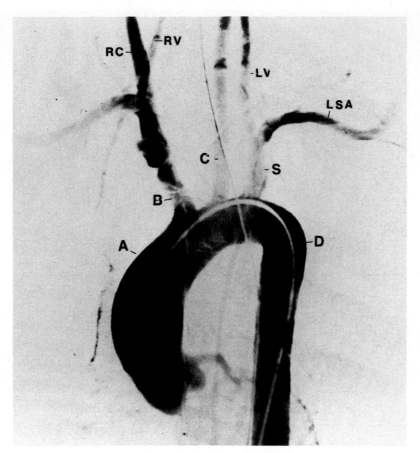

Figure 9.13. Normal aortogram. Contrast that was injected into the ascending aorta *A* shows the three major vessels and their branches coming off the arch. *B*, brachiocephalic artery; *C*, left common carotid; *D*, descending aorta; *LSA*, left subclavian artery; *LV*, left vertebral artery; *RC*, right common carotid; *RSA*, right subclavian artery; *RV*, right vertebral artery; *S*, left subclavian artery (aortic take-off).

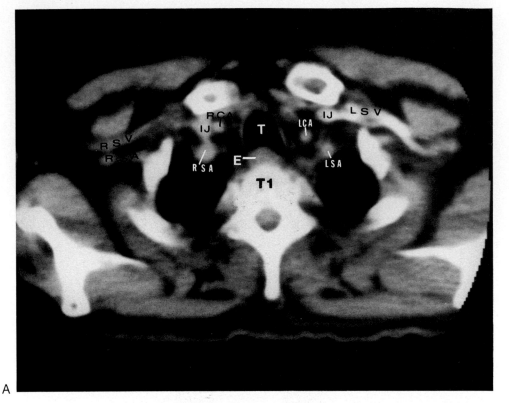

A

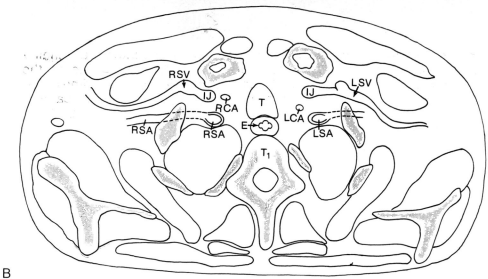

B

Figure 9.14. A and **B.** Section above the level of the bifurcation of the brachio-cephalic artery. The right subclavian artery *(RSA)* and the right carotid artery *(RCA)* are in the same anatomical position as the left subclavian artery *(LSA)* and left carotid artery *(LCA)*. The internal jugular veins *(IJ)*, which are usually anterior to the carotid arteries, are seen on both sides. The left subclavian vein *(LSV)* and right subclavian vein *(RSV)* are generally seen as the most anterior vascular structures. The esophagus *(E)* lies between the thoracic vertebral body *(T₁)* and the trachea *(T)*.

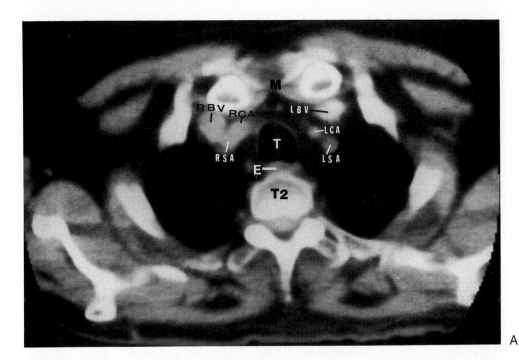

A

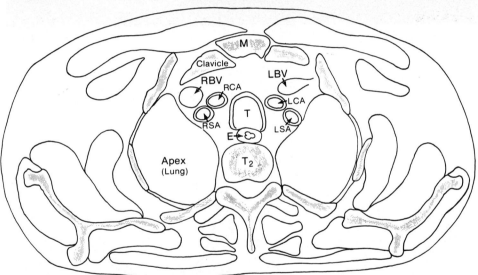

B

Figure 9.15. A and **B.** The right subclavian artery *(RSA)* and right carotid artery *(RCA)* are visualized at the bifurcation. Note that the left carotid artery *(LCA)* and left subclavian artery *(LSA)* are still in the same anatomical position as the previous slice. The right *(RBV)* and left *(LBV)* brachiocephalic veins are slightly anterolateral to the carotid arteries. *E,* esophagus; *M,* manubrium; *T,* trachea; *T₂,* thoracic vertebral body.

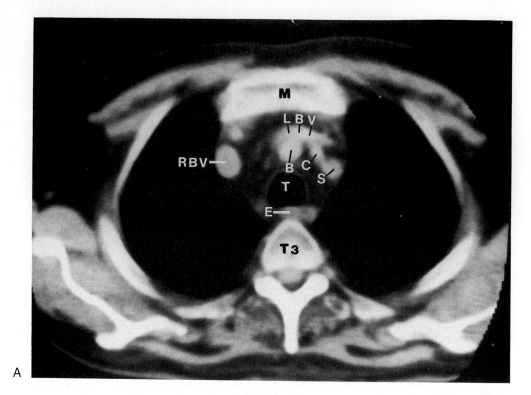

A

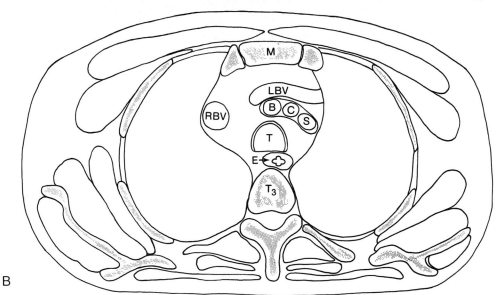

B

Figure 9.16. A and **B.** At this level five vessels can be routinely identified. Of these five, three are major branches of the aortic arch centrally located near the trachea, the brachiocephalic artery *(B)*, left carotid artery *(C)*, and left subclavian artery *(S)*. The left brachiocephalic veins *(LBV)* are seen coming across between the three major branches and the manubrium *(M)*. It will eventually join the right brachiocephalic vein *(RBV)* to form the superior vena cava. *E,* esophagus; *T,* trachea; T_3, thoracic vertebral body.

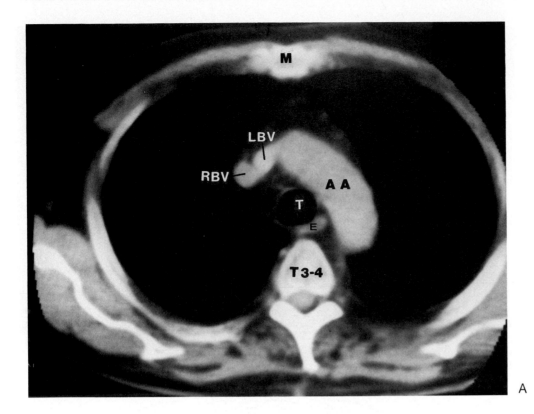

A

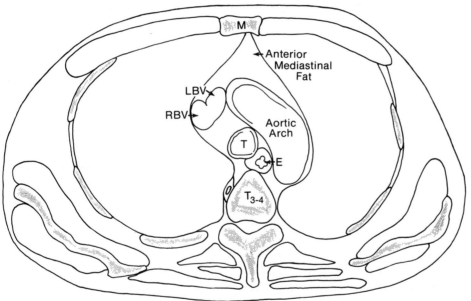

B

Figure 9.17. **A** and **B.** This section is through the aortic arch *(AA)*, which has a banana-shaped appearance. The right *(RBV)* and left *(LBV)* brachiocephalic veins are lateral to the aortic arch, forming the superior vena cava. Note the anterior and middle mediastinal fat, which is a low-attenuation homogeneous density that has an attenuation value of approximately −50 to −100 Hounsfield units *(HU)*. *E*, esophagus; *M*, manubrium; *T*, trachea. T_{3-4}, intervertebral disc.

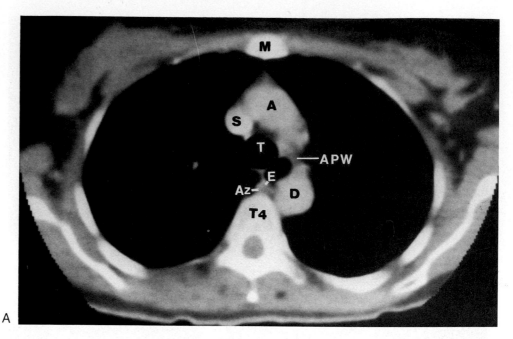

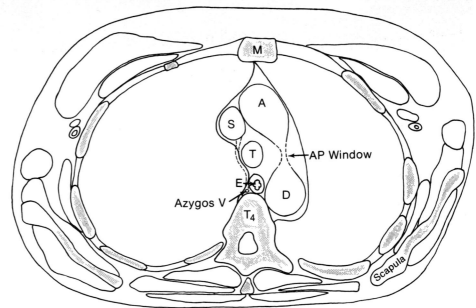

Figure 9.18. A and **B.** In this section below the aortic arch, the aortopulmonary window *(APW)* is seen between the ascending *(A)* and descending *(D)* aorta. The aortopulmonary window is formed by a portion of the aorta crossing over the main pulmonary artery. The azygos vein *(AZ)*, which provides venous drainage, is seen on the anterior side of the thoracic body *(T₄)*. It courses along the right side of the trachea *(T)* and drains into the superior vena cava *(S)*. *E,* esophagus; *M,* manubrium.

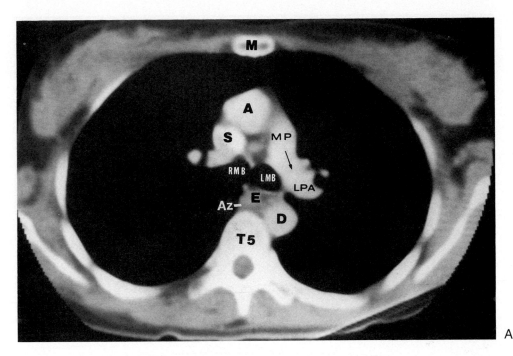

A

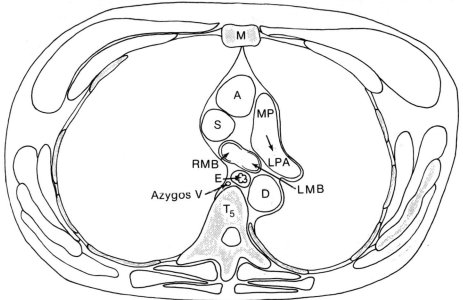

B

Figure 9.19. A and **B.** This section at the level of the carina shows the bifurcation of the right *(RMB)* and left *(LMB)* main stem bronchi. Generally, the main pulmonary artery *(MP)*, left pulmonary artery *(LPA)*, and right pulmonary artery (not seen here) appear as an inverted, Y-shaped structure. In this case, only the left pulmonary artery is seen branching from the main pulmonary artery, coursing posteriorly and slightly left to form the left lateral margin of the mediastinum. The ascending aorta *(A)* is the most anterior mediastinal structure seen, and the descending aorta *(D)* the most posterolateral mediastinal structure. *E*, esophagus; *T₅*, thoracic vertebral body; *M,* manubrium; *S,* superior vena cava; *Az;* azygos vein.

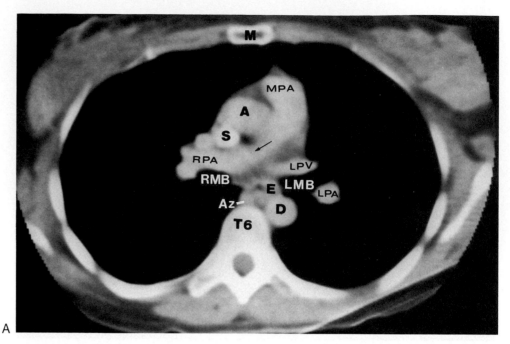

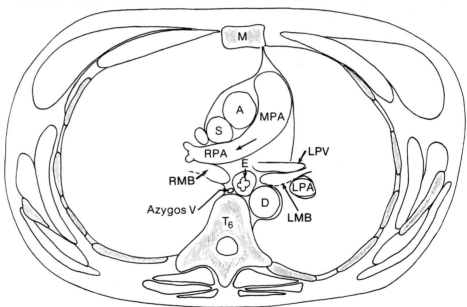

Fig. 9.20. A and **B.** This level, below the carina, shows the main pulmonary artery *(MPA)* branching *(arrow)* into the right pulmonary artery *(RPA)*. An inferior portion of the left pulmonary artery *(LPA)* is seen forming the inverted Y-shaped structure. Note the separated portion of the left pulmonary artery *(LPA)*, which has already crossed the left main stem bronchus and is coursing inferiorly. This structure should not be confused with a hilar mass. The superior vena cava *(S)* is between the ascending aorta *(A)* and the right pulmonary artery *(RPA)*. *Az*, azygos vein; *D*, descending aorta; *E*, esophagus; *LMB*, left main bronchus; *LPV*, left pulmonary vein; *M*, manubrium; *RMB*, right main bronchus; T_6, thoracic vertebral body.

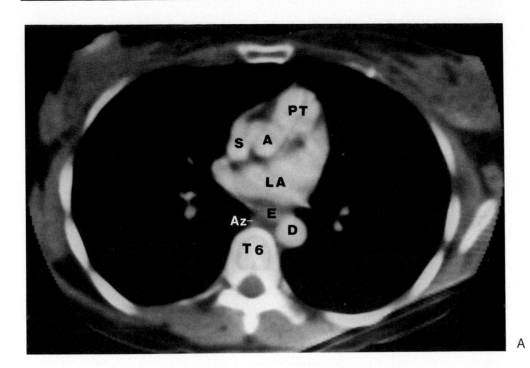

A

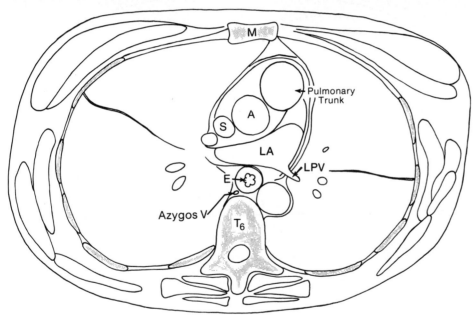

B

Figure 9.21. A and **B.** In this section, part of the pulmonary trunk *(PT)* is seen, and the left atrium *(LA)* is sandwiched between the ascending *(A)* and descending *(D)* aorta. Note that the ascending aorta is no longer the most anterior mediastinal structure seen. *E,* esophagus; *LPV,* left pulmonary vein; *S,* superior vena cava; *T₆,* thoracic vertebral body; *Az,* azygos vein.

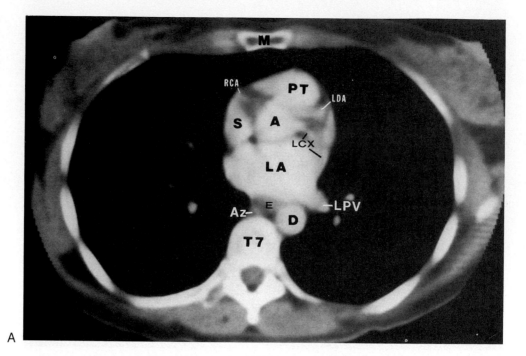

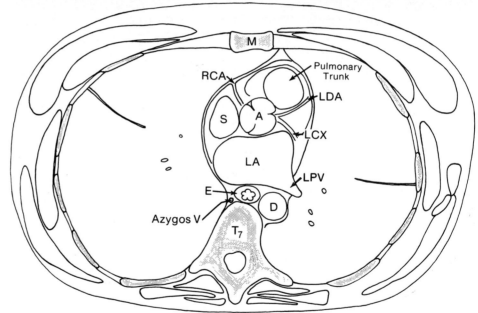

Figure 9.22. A and **B.** This section, at T₇ thoracic vertebral body, the beginning of the pulmonary trunk *(PT)* is seen arising from the right ventricle. The left atrium *(LA)* is seen sandwiched between the ascending *(A)* and the descending *(D)* aorta. The right coronary artery *(RCA)*, left circumflex coronary artery *(LCX)*, and left descending coronary artery *(LDA)* are seen coming off the ascending aorta. *Az,* azygos vein; *E,* esophagus; *M,* manubrium; *S,* superior vena cava; *LPV,* left pulmonary vein.

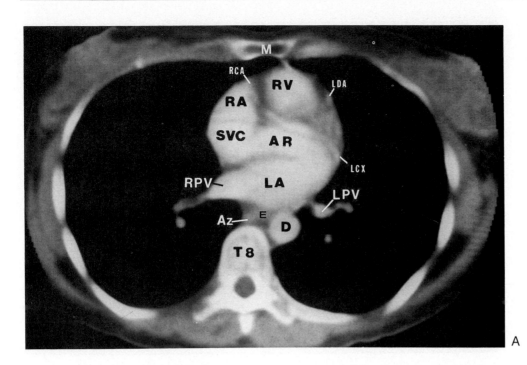

A

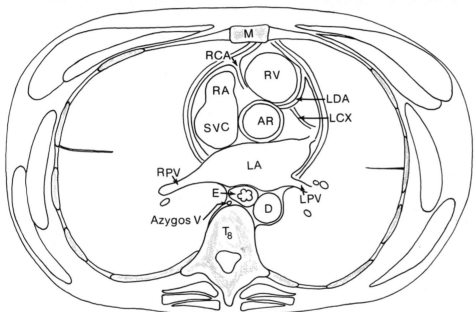

B

Figure 9.23. A and **B.** In this section the right *(RPV)* and the left *(LPV)* pulmonary veins are entering the left atrium *(LA)*. Again, the right coronary artery *(RCA)*, left descending coronary artery *(LDA)*, and left circumflex *(LCX)* are seen extending off the aortic root *(AR)*, which is the bottom of the aorta. Note that the superior vena cava *(SVC)* has entered the superior portion of the right atrium *(RA)*. D, descending aorta; E, esophagus; *LPV*, left pulmonary vein; *M*, manubrium; *T₈*, thoracic vertebral body; *Az*, azygos vein; *RV*, right ventricle.

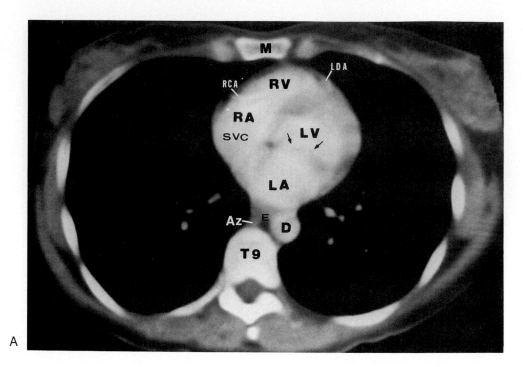

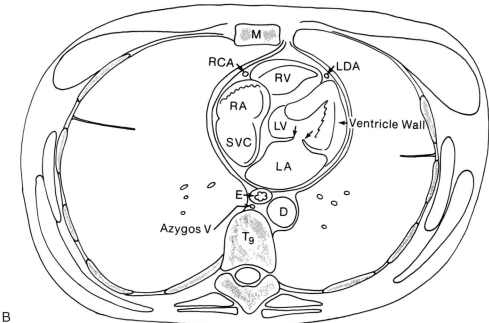

Figure 9.24. A and **B.** At this level, all four chambers of the heart can be seen. The arrows pointing between the left ventricle *(LV)* and the left atrium *(LA)* demonstrate the approximate area of the mitral valve. The right ventricle *(RV)*, seen as the most anterior vascular structure, is surrounded laterally by the right coronary artery *(RCA)* and the left descending coronary artery *(LDA)*. *Az,* azygos vein; *D,* descending aorta; *E,* esophagus; *M,* manubrium; *RA,* right atrium; *SVC,* superior vena cava; *T₉,* thoracic vertebral body.

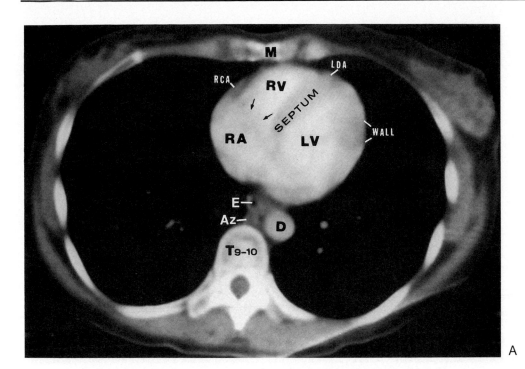

A

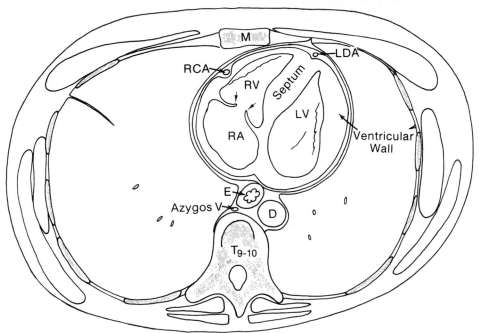

B

Figure 9.25. A and **B.** In this section, the *arrows* in the middle of the right ventricle *(RV)* and the right atrium *(RA)* point to the area of the tricuspid valve. Note the interventricular septum, which is separating the right *(RV)* and left *(LV)* ventricles. *Az,* azygos vein; *D,* descending aorta, *E,* esophagus; *LDA,* left descending coronary artery; *M,* manubrium; *RCA,* right coronary artery; *T₉₋₁₀,* intervertebral disc space.

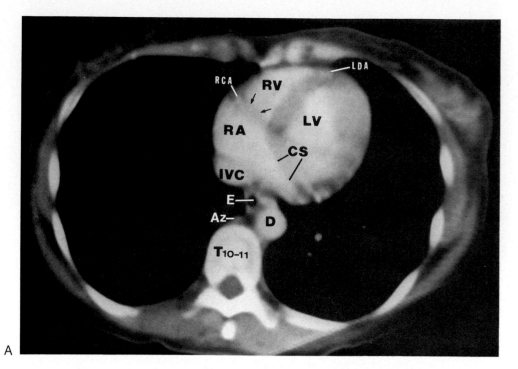

A

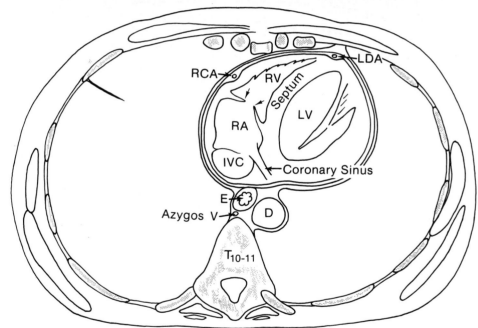

B

Figure 9.26. A and **B.** In this section the coronary sinus *(CS)*, which is the main venous drainage for the cardiac muscle, is adjacent to the inferior vena cava *(IVC)* and draining into the right atrium *(RA)*. Note the arrows pointing to the area of the tricuspid valve. Note also that the left ventricular *(LV)* wall is thicker than the right ventricular *(RV)* wall. *Az*, azygos vein; *D*, descending aorta; *E*, esophagus; *LDA*, left descending coronary artery; *RCA*, right coronary artery; T_{10-11}, intervertebral disc space.

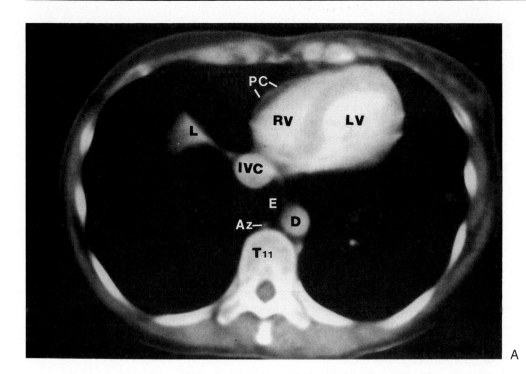

A

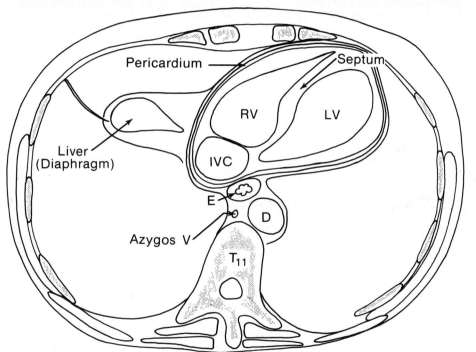

B

Figure 9.27. A and **B.** At this level through the base of the heart, only the right ventricle *(RV)*, left ventricle *(LV)*, septum, inferior vena cava *(IVC)*, and descending aorta *(D)* can be seen. The dome of the liver *(L)* and the pericardium *(PC)* are also visualized. *Az,* azygos vein; *E,* esophagus; *T₁₁,* thoracic vertebral body.

References and Suggested Readings

1. Barek L, Lautin R, Ledor S, et al. Role of CT in the assessment of superior vena caval obstruction. *J Comput Tomogr* 1982;6:121–126.
2. Baron RL, Levitt RG, Sagel SS, et al. Computed tomography in the evaluation of mediastinal widening. *Radiology* 1981;138:107–113.
3. Claussen CD, Bansjer D, Pfretsjschner C, et al. Bolus geometry and dynamics after intravenous contrast medium injection. *Radiology* 1984;153:365–368.
4. Godwin JD, Webb WR. Dynamic computed tomography in the evaluation of vascular lung lesions. *Radiology* 1981;138:629–635.
5. Grenier P, Valeyre D, Cluzel P, et al. Chronic diffuse interstitial lung disease: diagnostic value of chest radiography and high-resolution CT. *Radiology* 1991;179:123–132.
6. Glazer HS, Anderson DJ, DiCroce JJ, et al. Anatomy of the major fissure: evaluation with standard and thin-section CT. *Radiology* 1991;180:839–844.
7. Glazer HS, Molina PL, Siegel MJ, et al. High-attenuation mediastinal masses on unenhanced CT. *Am J Roetgenol* 1991;156:45–60.
8. Heitzman ER. Computed tomography of the thorax: current perspectives. *Am J Roetgenol* 1981;136:2–12.
9. Kaye AD, Janssen R, Arger PH, et al. Mediastinal computed tomography in myasthenia gravis. *J Comput Tomogr* 1983;7:273–279.
10. Kormano MJ, Dean PB, Hamlin DJ. Upper extremity contrast medium infusion in computed tomography of upper mediastinal masses. *J Comput Assist Tomogr* 1980;4:617–620.
11. Littleton JT, Durizch ML, Moeller G, et al. Pulmonary masses: contrast enhancement. *Radiology* 1990;177:861–871.
12. Mathieson JR, Mayo JR, Staples CA, et al. Chronic diffuse infiltrative lung disease: comparison of diagnostic accuracy of CT and chest radiography. *Radiology* 1989;171:111–16.
13. Mayo JR, Webb WR, Gould R, et al. High-resolution CT of the lungs: an optimal approach. *Radiology* 1987;163:507–510.
14. McCarthy S, Moss AA. The use of a flow rate injectors for contrast-enhanced computed tomography. *Radiology* 1984;151:800.
15. Micklos JJ, Proto AV. CT demonstration of the coronary sinus. *J Comput Assist Tomgr* 1985;9:60–64.
16. Muller NL. Clinical value of high-resolution CT in chronic diffuse lung disease. *AJR* 1991;157:1163–1170.
17. Murata K, Kan A, Rojas KA, et al. Optimization of computed tomography: technique to demonstrate the fine structure of the lung. *Invest Radiol* 1988;23:170–175.
18. Naidich DP, Zeerhouni EA, Siegelman SS. *Computed tomography of the thorax.* New York: Raven, 1984.
19. Proto AV, Thomas SR. Pulmonary nodules studied by computed tomography. *Radiology* 1985;156:149–153.
20. Robbins AH, Pugatch RD, Gerzof SG, et al. Further observations on the medical efficacy of computed tomography of the chest and abdomen. *Radiology* 1980;137:719–725.
21. Robinson PJ, Kreel L. Pulmonary tissue attenuation with computed tomography: comparison of inspiration and expiration scans. *Comput Assist Tomogr* 1979;3:740–748.
22. Rosenblum LJ, Mauceri RA, Wellenstein DE, et al. Density patterns in the normal lung as determined by computed tomography. *Radiology* 1980;137:409–416.
23. Shipley RT, McLoud TC, Dedrick CG, et al. Computed tomography of the tracheal bronchus. *J Comput Assist Tomogr* 1985;9:53–55.
24. Sones PJ, Torres WE, Colvin RS, et al. Effectiveness of CT in evaluating intrathoracic masses. *Am J Roetgenol* 1982;139:469–475.
25. Swensen SJ, Aughenbaugh GL, Douglas WW, et al. High-resolution CT of the lungs: Findings in various pulmonary diseases. *Am J Roetgenol* 1992;158:971–979.

Abdomen and Pelvis

Positioning

Abdominal and pelvic examinations are usually done in the supine position with the patient's arms above the head. For a full examination a posterior–anterior (PA) localizer is obtained, with scanning starting at the xiphoid process and continuing to the symphysis pubis. If the area of interest is in the upper abdomen, scanning starts at the xiphoid process and continues to the iliac crest. If the pelvis is of clinical interest, scanning starts at the iliac crest and continues to the symphysis pubis.

Occasionally prone and decubitus positions are used when indicated.

Technique

A 10-mm slice thickness is commonly used for abdominal and pelvic examinations. The parameter for couch indexing varies, depending on the clinical history and the area to be examined. Couch indexes of 10, 15, and 20 mm are used for abdominal and pelvic examinations. We suggest 10 mm for these examinations because we believe that a larger couch index does not give the firm, detailed diagnosis that is needed by clinicians. In certain instances, small parameters (5–8 mm) may be needed for localization of small lesions or for specific organs such as the pancreas or the kidney.

Short exposure times (1–3 sec) are needed for routine examinations, particularly in the abdomen where respiratory and peristaltic motion can degrade image quality. Frequently these exposure times need to be increased to reduce beam hardening commonly found at the inferior portion of the ilium, the femoral heads, and the bladder, which may be filled with injected iodinated contrast (Fig. 10.1). Patients with large hips also present problems with artifact as a result of underpenetration.

In order to get optimal diagnostic images in abdominal and pelvic scanning, suspended respiration is essential. When performing these examina-

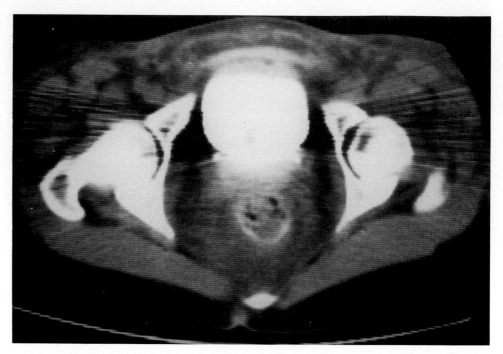

Figure 10.1. Streaking artifact resulting from beam hardening.

tions, it is particularly important that the patient hold his or her breath the same way for each slice. Anatomical fluctuation can easily occur with inconsistent breathing owing to the diaphragm compressing differently on abdominal organs. We have found suspended respiration at resting volume to be the procedure of choice in these examinations.

Contrast Enhancement

OPACIFICATION OF THE ALIMENTARY TRACT

Use of contrast to opacify the alimentary tract is mandatory for precise CT examinations. Good opacification of the alimentary tract prevents such difficulties as confusing unopacified loops of bowel such as the duodenum for a mass at the head of the pancreas, or confusing other parts of the bowel for lymph nodes or abscesses.

Dilute barium sulfate suspensions and water-soluble solutions (diatrizoate meglumine and diatrizoate sodium) are the most common positive contrast agents used for abdominal and pelvic CT scans.

BARIUM SULFATE SUSPENSIONS

There are many flavored, low-concentration barium suspensions on the market specifically for abdominal and pelvic CT. Generally, barium sulfate suspensions are economical, effective, and easily administered, and they have a flavor acceptable to most patients.

Because barium sulfate is not water-soluble, it should not be used with patients suspected of having gastrointestinal perforation. Leakage of barium sulfate into the abdominal and pelvic cavities can lead to severe complications such as peritonitis or peritoneal adhesions. It should not be used in patients going to surgery who are hypersensitive to it or have a bowel obstruction.

With barium sulfate suspension, it is important to perform examinations as close to manufacturer's specified time as possible. Waiting too long after the preparation has been ingested allows too much water to be absorbed by the bowel, leaving dense residual barium, which can cause streaking artifact.

Water-Soluble Contrast Agents

The availability of water-soluble contrast agents has created an invaluable alternative to barium sulfate solutions, especially in cases such as gastrointestinal perforation where barium sulfate cannot be used. Water-soluble solutions give a good coating and have a fast transit time because of their ability to increase peristaltic stimulation. However, if long exposure times (5 sec or more) are going to be used, peristaltic stimulation is considered a disadvantage because of motion artifact.

When using water-soluble solutions, extreme care must be exercised during preparation of the solution. Diatrizoate solutions of 15% to 40% are considered clinically hypertonic and may draw extreme amounts of fluid into the intestine, which could lead to hypovolemia. Particular attention must be paid to young or debilitated children and to elderly persons suffering from malnutrition and general ill health. In such cases, dehydration is likely to already be a problem. Diatrizoate preparations at concentrations of 2% to 5% have been found to be clinically effective. Other adverse reactions include nausea, vomiting, and slight diarrhea, especially when water-soluble agents are used in large volumes or in high concentrations. In a few patients urticaria (hives) has occurred.

Suggested Contrast Preparation Volumes for Abdominal/Pelvic Scanning (Water-Soluble and Barium Sulfate Solutions)

Upper abdomen only: 400–600 ml orally 15–30 min before scan; 300 ml oral immediately before scan; patient in right decubitus position 3–5 min.

Abdomen and pelvis (oral and by enema): 700–900 ml orally 30–45 min before scan; 800–1,000 ml enema immediately before scan; 300 ml orally immediately before scan; patient in right decubitus position 3–5 min.

Abdomen and pelvis (oral only): 1,200–1,500 ml 45–60 min before scan; 300 ml immediately before scan; patient in right decubitus position 3–5 min.

Pelvis only: 700–900 ml orally 30–45 min before scan; 800–1,000 ml enema immediately before scan.

If patients are unable to drink the oral contrast agent because of nausea and vomiting, nasal gastric tubes should be used to introduce the solution.

PREEXAMINATION REGIMEN

The night before an abdominal or pelvic examination, the patient should take a laxative. Fecal material can appear as a mass on CT and restricts the flow of contrast. Its removal improves coating of the bowel wall and promotes faster movement of oral contrast. Before the examination, the patient must not have any solid food, as such material can simulate a gastric tumor. Below is a suggested regimen for patients prior to abdominal and pelvic examinations.

MORNING SCAN

Clear liquid supper the night before
Laxative to clean the small and large bowel
Nothing by mouth after midnight

AFTERNOON SCAN

Clear liquid supper the night before
Laxative to clean the small and large bowel
Clear liquid breakfast
Nothing by mouth after breakfast

EVENING SCAN

Clear liquid supper the night before
Laxative to clean the small and large bowel
Clear liquids for breakfast and lunch
Nothing by mouth after lunch

ALIMENTARY TRACT OPACIFICATION PROBLEMS

There are several specific problems related to the contrast used for opacification of the alimentary tract. The most common problem is inadequate opacification of the C-loop of the duodenum. If this area is not adequately opacified, it can be mistakenly read as a pancreatic mass (Fig. 10.2). To help overcome this problem, the patient should drink approximately 300 ml of the oral contrast agent and then roll into a right decubitus position for 3–5 min immediately before the examination begins. This allows the contrast to empty rapidly from the stomach into the duodenum. In other portions of the small bowel, which may be unopacified, repeat scanning is necessary after additional oral contrast. If the colon is not completely opacified in cases where only oral contrast is administered, an enema may be required, particularly in the pelvic area.

INTRAVENOUS CONTRAST ENHANCEMENT

Intravenous (IV) contrast is important in the evaluation of abdominal and pelvic vascular structures such as the portal vein, inferior vena cava, abdominal aorta, and iliac arteries and veins. Lesions can be characterized

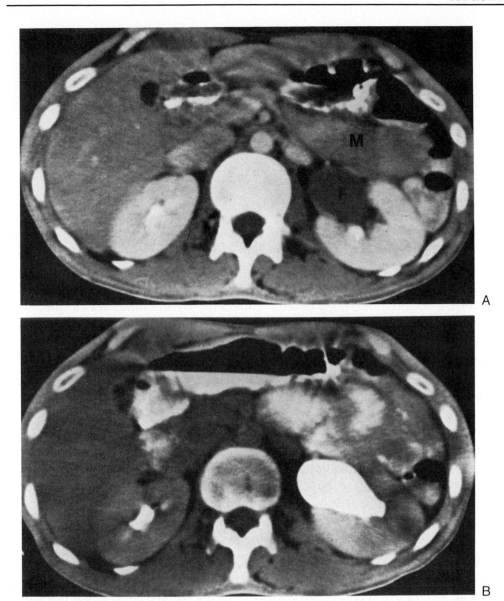

Figure 10.2. A and **B.** Pseudotumor of the pancreas. Initial scan **(A)** shows a soft tissue mass *(M)* in the tail of the pancreas and a fluid mass *(F)* in the left renal pelvis. Delayed scan **(B)** after administration of additional oral contrast shows the mass in the tail of the pancreas to be loops of jejunum. The large extra-renal pelvis is also filled with IV contrast.

and identified by the way they enhance or by their attenuation when compared to normally enhanced surrounding tissue. Intravenous contrast media are also important in visualizing the ureters and bladder. The methods of IV contrast administration are: (1) single bolus injection; (2) drip infusion; (3) bolus injection, then drip infusion; (4) drip infusion, then bolus injection; and (5) multiple bolus injections.

Although these are the same methods used for chest CT, the timing is significantly different: A longer delay is needed for media circulation (Table 10.1). Approximately 30 sec is needed for iodine to complete antecubital vein to portal circulation. The dilution of iodine is much more rapid because it mixes with a greater blood volume and there is extravascular diffusion to surrounding tissue (20).

Table 10.1. *Approximate normal circulation time for contrast to arrive in abdominal vessels after antecubital vein injection*

Abdominal vessel	Approximate normal circulation time (sec)
Abdominal aorta	14
Renal artery	15
Hepatic arteries	16
Portal veins	30

Ideally, IV contrast injections for abdominal and pelvic examinations are made through an 18-gauge catheter at the antecubital fossa of the right arm (see Contrast Enhancement, Chapter 9). Injections into the leg or foot should always be avoided because of the possibility of thrombophlebitis. Contrast injected into a leg or foot, especially by the bolus technique, can produce streaking artifact at the inferior vena cava because of the rapid accumulation and lack of diffusion of the contrast owing to the unidirectional flow.

SINGLE BOLUS INJECTION

A single bolus injection of 60–100 ml of contrast medium gives immediate intravascular opacification that lasts 20–40 sec. After this time, the contrast medium begins to diffuse into the extravascular space, giving organ tissue opacification. Effective opacification lasts 1–2 min. This method works well when a specific area is in question and is examined by dynamic scanning without table indexing.

DRIP INFUSION

The drip infusion technique is an alternative when access to an antecubital vein is not possible. Because inconsistent flow rates are a major problem with drip infusion (see Drip Infusion, Chapter 9), this technique is avoided when vascular enhancement is of primary interest. When using this technique, a scan and process mode should be used with scanning starting 3–5 min after the infusion has begun. After infusion is complete, a rapid mode may be used if desired.

BOLUS FOLLOWED BY DRIP INFUSION

Bolus injection followed by drip infusion gives a longer maintained plasma iodine level. The initial 30-ml bolus achieves the elevated plasma iodine level, which is followed by an 150-ml rapid drip infusion; to help maintain the iodine level. Scanning begins 1 min after the start of the drip infusion to allow filling of hepatic vasculature and tissue. Because the plasma iodine level is maintained longer (10–15 min), this technique is used for routine examinations. However, after this time period, there is a gradual drop in opacification. The bolus followed by drip infusion method is widely accepted because of its convenience.

DRIP INFUSION FOLLOWED BY BOLUS INJECTION

Drip infusion and the bolus injection is used when there is a specific area of interest such as the pancreas or the kidneys. A 150-ml rapid drip infusion allows diffusion of contrast to the organ tissue. Once the area of interest is reached, the bolus is administered. The timing of rapid scanning depends on the area of interest (see Table 10.1). Administration of the bolus elevates the plasma iodine concentration, resulting in excellent vascular and tissue opacification.

MULTIPLE-BOLUS INJECTION (CT ANGIOGRAPHY)

Multiple-bolus injection is most commonly associated with computed tomography angiography (CTA). CTA is invaluable when examining and evaluating abdominal vascularity. Portal hypertension, dissecting aneurysms, and the tumor's relationship to vascular structures can be better defined with CTA (3,10,20,40).

For CTA examinations we recommend 360° scan rotation angle, 95 mA, and an exposure time of 1–3 sec. The exposure time varies depending on patient size. With scanning starting in the low (20%) heat unit range and using a 10-mm slice thickness and couch index, 13–16 slices can be obtained before excessive heat units accumulate. These are enough slices to cover major abdominal vascular structures.

Multiple-bolus injection for CTA scanning differs slightly from the similar technique used in chest scanning (see Multiple Bolus Injection, Chapter 9). The most important point that must be made is that CTA scanning begins much later after the initial bolus. Because 80% of the blood supply to the liver is via the portal system, scanning begins 30 sec (for the average normal antecubital vein to portal circulation, (Table 10.1) after the start of the initial bolus of 30–40 ml of contrast. In patients who have a history of portal hypertension or chronic heart failure, a longer waiting period (1 min) is necessary. Enhancement is sustained by an additional 10–15 ml of contrast medium administered by a power injector set at a flow rate of 5–7 ml/sec; if no power injector is available, the contrast is administered continuously by hand at approximately the same rate.

USE OF A TAMPON FOR VAGINAL ENHANCEMENT

Use of a tampon is an excellent and easy way for negative (air) enhancement of the vagina (6). Its insertion results in dilation and entrapment of air. This simple procedure is helpful for easier anatomical localization.

USE OF GAS FOR BLADDER ENHANCEMENT

A negative contrast agent (carbon dioxide) has proved to be advantageous for the assessment of intravesicular tumors (12,32). The main advantage over iodinated contrast medium is that the gas does not overshadow these tumors, as the high density of iodinated medium is likely to do. This allows easier assessment of the tumor's true size. Carbon dioxide is used instead of air to prevent a rare but possible air embolism (32).

For demonstration of intravesicular tumors by a negative contrast agent, a Foley catheter is inserted into the bladder and intravenous contrast is drained. Carbon dioxide is introduced into the bladder by the Foley catheter until the patient has a feeling of fullness. The catheter is then clamped. After instillation of the gas, the patient is scanned in either the prone or the supine position. The position used is governed by the location of the lesion.

NORMAL ANATOMY OF THE ABDOMEN

The series of abdominal CT images in Figs. 10.3 through 10.13 were obtained at 95 mA, an exposure time of 3.4 sec, a 398° scan angle, and a couch index and slice thickness of 10 mm. For intravenous contrast enhancement a drip/bolus method was used.

The series of abdominal computed tomography angiograms (CTA), found in Figs. 10.14 through 10.22 were obtained using an abdominal CTA protocol (95 mA, exposure time 3.0 sec, 360° scan angle) with the multiple-bolus method for intravenous contrast enhancement. A slice thickness and couch index of 10 mm was used.

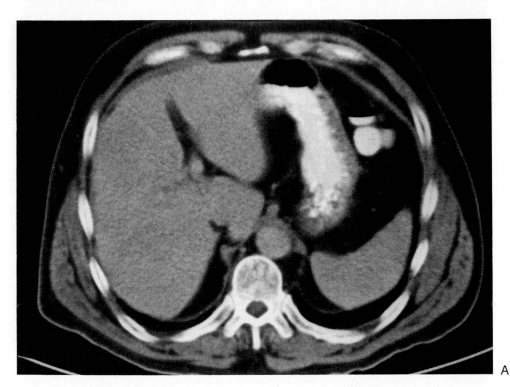

A

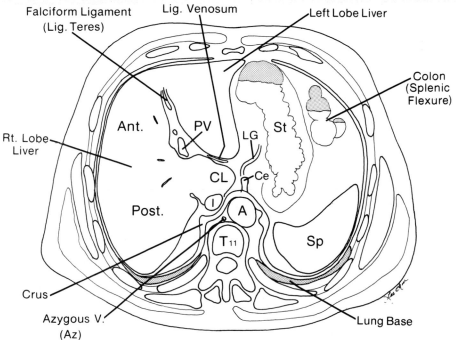

B

Figure 10.3. A and **B.** This section, approximately at the xiphoid process, shows the falciform ligament inside the fissure of ligamentum teres. The falciform ligament is a fold of peritoneum that helps attach the liver to the diaphragm. *A,* aorta; *Ant.,* anterior segment right lobe of liver; *Az,* azygous vein; *Ce,* celiac artery; *CL,* caudate lobe; *I,* inferior vena cava; *LG,* left gastric artery; *Post.,* posterior segment, right lobe of liver; *PV,* portal vein; *Sp,* spleen; *St,* stomach.

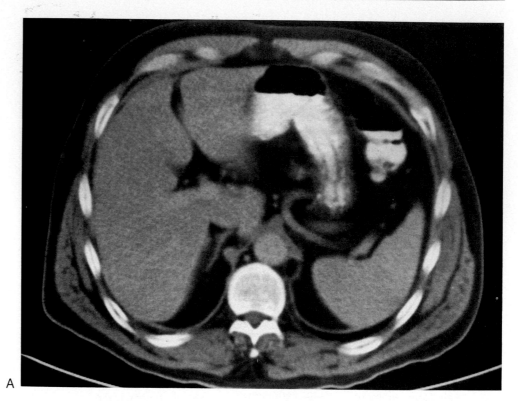

A

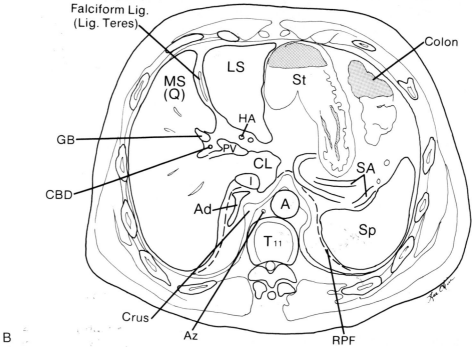

B

Figure 10.4. A and **B.** In this section, the fissure of the ligamentum teres is separating the lateral *(LS)* and medial *(MS)* segments of the left lobe of the liver. The medial segment is also known as the quadrate *(Q)* lobe. The *broken lines* represents the retroperitoneal fascia *(RPF),* which is an imaginary border that divides the abdomen into two compartments. Anything ventral to this line is in the intra-abdominal compartment; anything dorsal is in the retroperitoneal compartment. *A,* aorta; *Ad,* adrenal gland; *Az,* azygous vein; *CBD,* common bile duct; *CL,* caudate lobe; *GB,* gallbladder; *HA,* hepatic artery; *I,* inferior vena cava; *PV,* portal vein; *SA,* splenic artery; *Sp,* spleen; *St,* stomach.

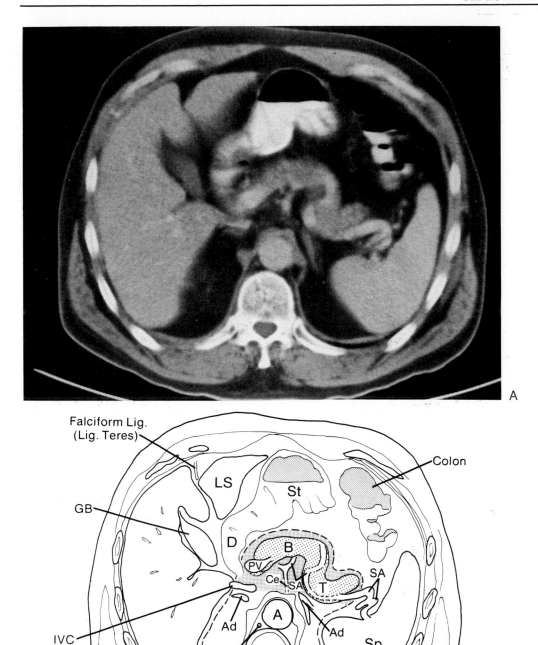

Fig. 10.5. A and **B.** Cross-section at the splenic hilus. *A*, aorta; *Ad*, adrenal gland; *Az*, azygous vein; *B*, pancreatic body; *Ce*, celiac artery; *D*, duodenum; *GB*, gallbladder; *IVC*, inferior vena cava; *LS*, lateral segment, left lobe of liver; *PV*, portal vein; *RPF*, retroperitoneal fascia; *SA*, splenic artery; *Sp*, spleen; *St*, stomach; *T*, pancreatic tail.

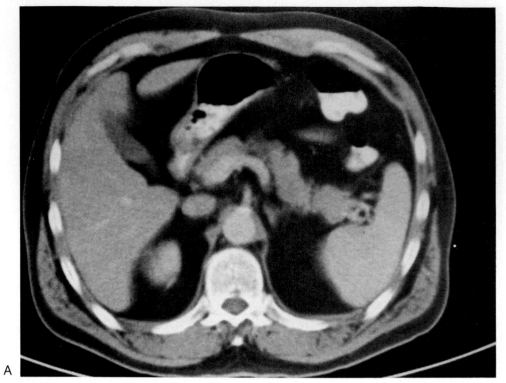

A

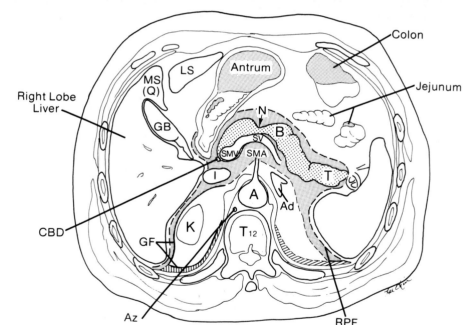

B

FIG. 10.6. A and **B.** Scan 2 cm caudal to the splenic hilus demonstrates the splenic vein *(SV)*, which runs posterior to the pancreas joining the superior mesenteric vein *(SMV)*. The splenic vein and superior mesenteric vein form the portal vein. *A*, aorta; *Ad*, adrenal gland; *Az*, azygous vein; *B*, pancreatic body; *CBD*, common bile duct; *GB*, gallbladder; *I*, inferior vena cava; *GF*, Gerota's fascia; *K*, kidney; *LS*, lateral segment, left lobe of liver; *MS(Q)*, medial segment, left lobe of liver (quadrate lobe); *N*, pancreatic neck, *RPF*, retroperitoneal fascia; *SMA*, superior mesenteric artery; *T*, pancreatic tail.

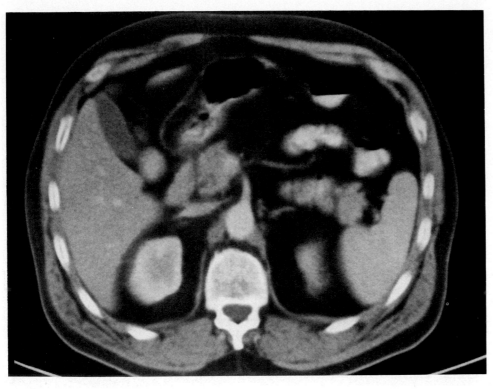

A

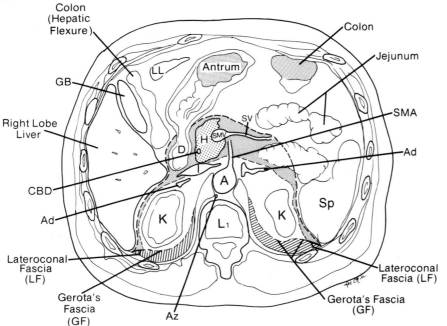

B

Figure 10.7. A and **B.** Section at the level of the second portion of the duodenum *(D)*. Note that the pancreatic head *(H)* is outlined by the duodenal C-loop. *A,* aorta; *Ad,* adrenal gland; *Az,* azygous vein; *CBD,* common bile duct; *GB,* gallbladder; *I,* inferior vena cava; *K,* kidney; *LL,* left lobe of liver; *SMA,* superior mesenteric artery; *SMV,* superior mesenteric vein; *Sp,* spleen; *SV,* splenic vein. *Fine dots,* anterior pararenal space; *white area,* perirenal space; *hatched area,* posterior pararenal space; *thick broken line,* retroperitoneal fascia.

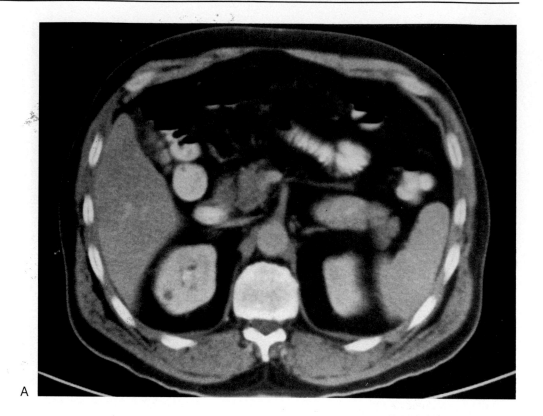

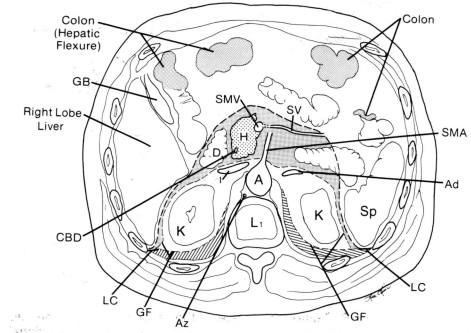

Figure 10.8. A and **B.** The retroperitoneum contains three compartments: the anterior and posterior pararenal spaces and the perirenal space. The anterior pararenal space *(fine dots)* contains the pancreas, duodenum *(D)*, and ascending and descending colon. The posterior pararenal space *(hatched area)* contains no organs. The perirenal space *(white area)* contains perirenal fat, adrenal glands *(Ad)*, ureters (not seen), and kidneys *(K)*. Gerota's fascia *(GF)* and lateroconal fascia *(LC)* delineate the anterior and posterior pararenal compartments. *A*, aorta; *Az*, azygous vein; *CBD*, common bile duct; *GB*, gallbladder; *I*, inferior vena cava; *SMA*, superior mesenteric artery; *SMV*, superior mesenteric vein; *Sp*, spleen; *SV*, splenic vein. *Thick broken line,* retroperitoneal fascia.

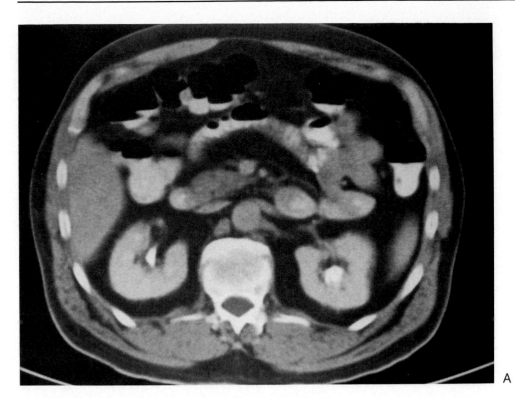

A

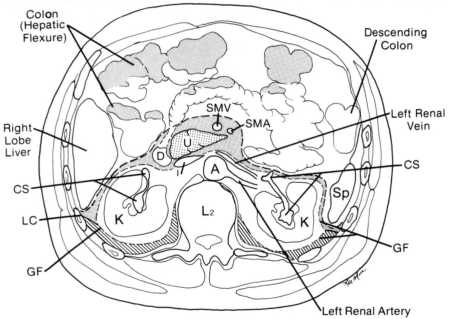

B

Figure 10.9. A and **B.** Scan taken at the level of the left renal hilus. The left renal artery is seen coming off the aorta *(A)*, and the larger left renal vein is coursing anterior to the renal artery. *CS,* collecting system; *D,* duodenum (second portion); *GF,* Gerota's fascia; *I,* inferior vena cava; *K,* kidney; *LC,* lateroconal fascia; *SMA,* superior mesenteric artery; *SMV,* superior mesenteric vein; *Sp,* spleen; *U,* uncinate process of pancreas. *Fine dots,* anterior pararenal space; *white area,* perirenal space; *hatched area,* posterior pararenal space; *thick broken line,* retroperitoneal fascia.

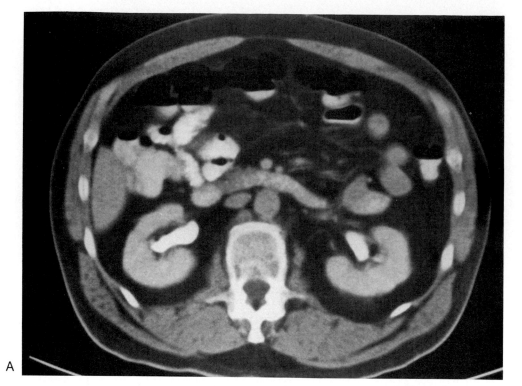

A

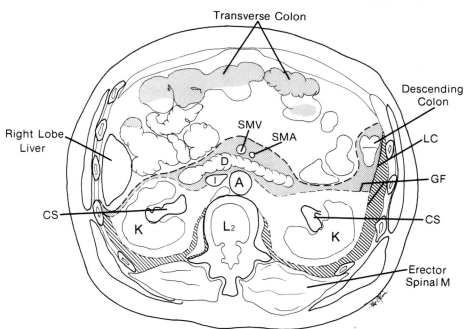

B

Figure 10.10. A and **B.** Scan taken at the level of the third portion of the duodenum *(D)*. Note that the superior mesenteric artery *(SMA)* and superior mesenteric vein *(SMV)* are anterior to the duodenum. *A,* aorta; *CS,* collecting system; *GF,* Gerota's fascia; *I,* inferior vena cava; *K,* kidney; *LC,* lateroconal fascia. *Fine dots,* anterior pararenal space; *white area,* perirenal space; *hatched area,* posterior pararenal space; *thick broken line,* retroperitoneal fascia.

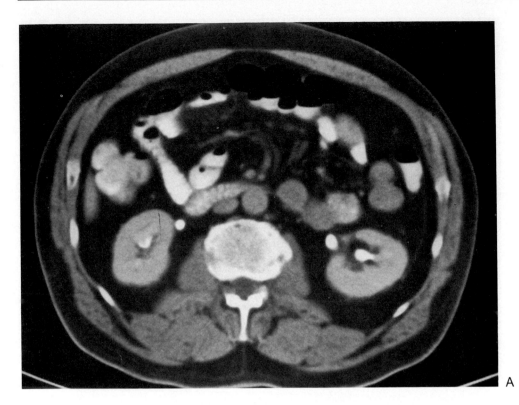

A

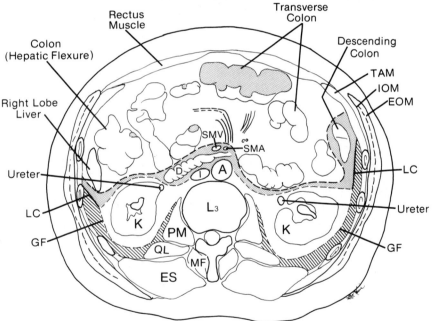

B

Figure 10.11. A and **B.** The transverse abdominal muscle *(TAM)* compresses
the abdominal viscera, the internal oblique muscle *(IOM)* and eternal oblique
muscle *(EOM)*, which also compress the abdominal viscera and allow flexing
and rotating of the vertebral column. The multifidus muscle *(MF)* assists in
rotation of the vertebral column. Flexing of the trunk is made possible by the
psoas muscle *(PM)* and quadratus lumborum muscle *(QL)*. The back muscles
are known as erector spinal muscle *(ES)*. *A*, aorta; *D*, duodenum (third portion); *GF*, Gerota's fascia; *I*, inferior vena cava; *K*, kidney; *LC*, lateroconal
fascia; *SMA*, superior mesenteric artery; *SMV*, superior mesenteric vein. *Fine
dots*, anterior pararenal space; *white area*, perirenal space; *hatched area*,
posterior pararenal space, *thick broken line*, retroperitoneal fascia.

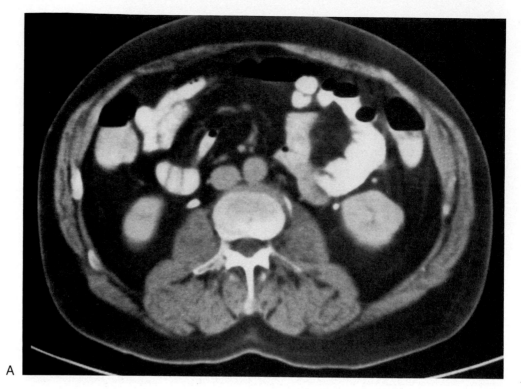

A

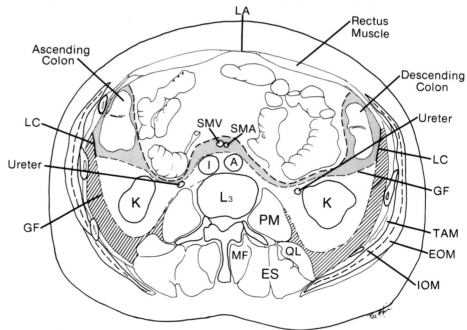

B

Figure 10.12. A and **B.** Scan taken at the lower poles of the kidneys *(K)*. The linea alba *(LA)* joins the paired rectus muscles. *A,* aorta; *EOM,* external oblique muscle; *ES,* erector spinal muscle; *GF,* Gerota's fascia; *I,* inferior vena cava; *IOM,* internal oblique muscle; *LC,* lateroconal fascia; *MF,* multifidus muscle; *PM,* psoas muscle; *QL,* quadratus lumborum muscle; *SMA,* superior mesenteric artery; *SMV,* superior mesenteric vein; *TAM,* transverse abdominal muscle. *Fine dots,* anterior pararenal space; *white area,* perirenal space; *hatched area,* posterior pararenal space; *thick broken line,* retroperitoneal fascia.

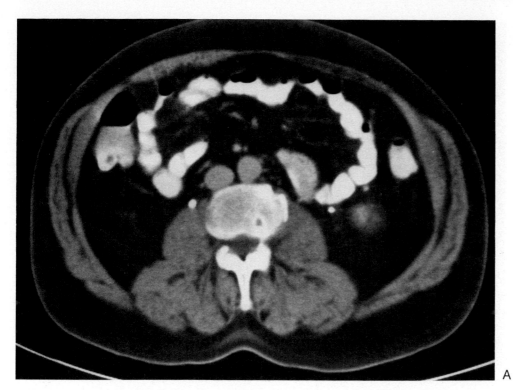

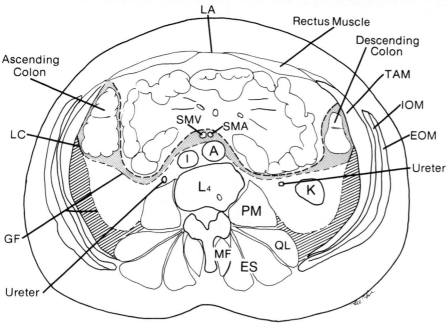

Figure 10.13. A and **B.** Scan taken at L₄ demonstrates only the inferior pole of the left kidney *(K)*; no other solid retroperitoneal or intra-abdominal organs are seen. *A,* aorta; *EOM,* external oblique muscle; *ES,* erector spinal muscle; *GF,* Gerota's fascia; *I,* inferior vena cava; *IOM,* internal oblique muscle; *LA,* linea alba; *LC,* lateroconal fascia; *MF,* multifidus muscle; *PM,* psoas muscle; *QL,* quadratus lumborum muscle; *SMA,* superior mesenteric artery; *SMV,* superior mesenteric vein; *TAM,* transverse abdominal muscle. *Fine dots,* anterior pararenal space; *white area,* perirenal space; *hatched area,* posterior pararenal space; *thick broken line,* retroperitoneal fascia.

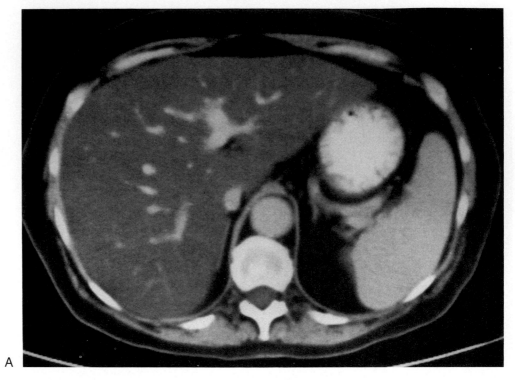

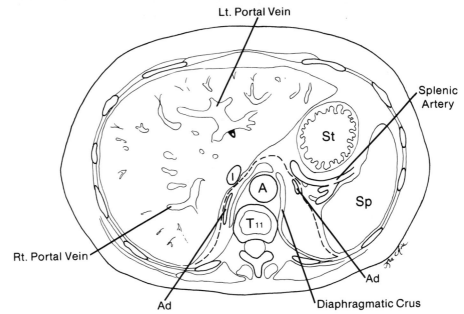

Figure 10.14. A and **B.** *A,* aorta; *Ad,* adrenal gland; *I,* inferior vena cava; *Sp,* spleen; *St,* stomach. *Thick broken line,* retroperitoneal fascia.

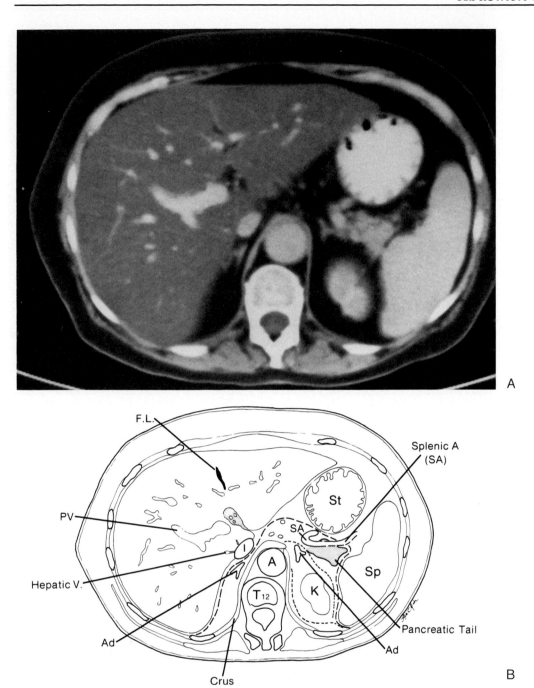

Figure 10.15. A and **B**. *A*, aorta; *Ad*, adrenal gland; *F.L.*, falciform ligament; *I*, inferior vena cava; *K*, kidney; *PV*, portal vein; *Sp*, spleen; *St*, stomach. *Thick broken line*, retroperitoneal fascia; *thin broken line*, Gerota's fascia; *solid line*, lateroconal fascia.

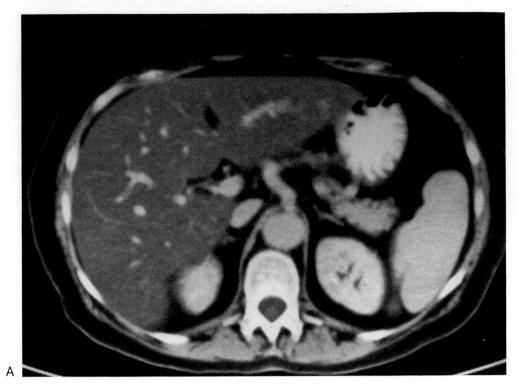

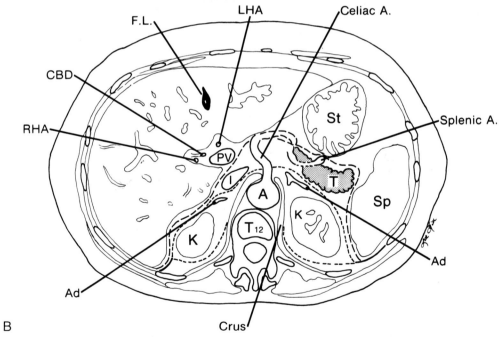

Figure 10.16. A and **B.** *A,* aorta; *Ad,* adrenal gland; *CBD,* common bile duct; *F.L.,* falciform ligament; *I,* inferior vena cava; *K,* kidney; *LHA,* left hepatic artery; *PV,* portal vein; *RHA,* right hepatic artery; *Sp,* spleen; *St,* stomach; *T,* pancreatic tail. *Thick broken line,* retroperitoneal fascia; *thin broken line,* Gerota's fascia; *solid line,* lateroconal fascia.

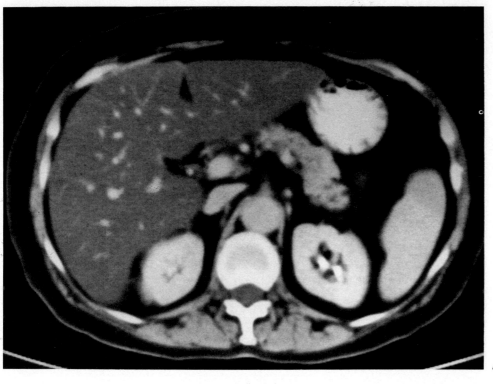

A

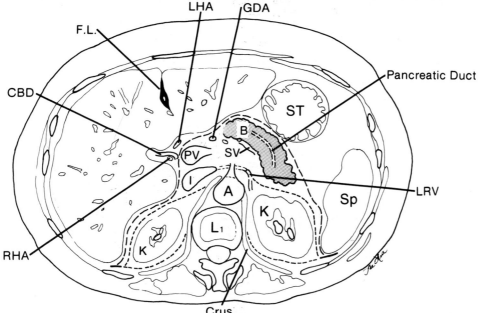

B

Figure 10.17. A and **B.** *A,* aorta; *B,* pancreatic body; *CBD,* common bile duct; *F.L.,* falciform ligament; *GDA,* gastroduodenal artery; *I,* inferior vena cava; *K,* kidney; *LHA,* left hepatic artery; *LRV,* left renal vein; *PV,* portal vein; *RHA,* right hepatic artery; *Sp,* spleen; *St,* stomach; *SV,* splenic vein. *Thick broken line,* retroperitoneal fascia; *thin broken line,* Gerota's fascia; *solid line,* lateroconal fascia.

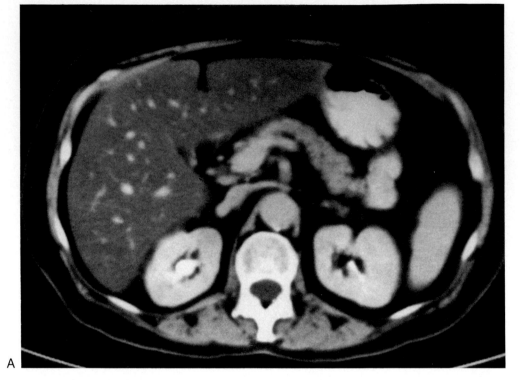

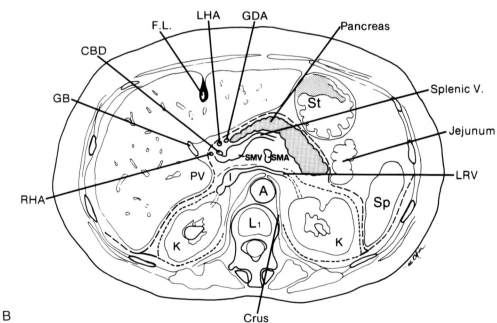

Figure 10.18. **A** and **B.** *A,* aorta; *CBD,* common bile duct; *F.L.,* falciform ligament; *GB,* gallbladder; *GDA,* gastroduodenal artery; *I,* inferior vena cava; *K,* kidney; *LHA,* left hepatic artery; *LRV,* left renal vein; *RHA,* right hepatic artery; *SMA,* superior mesenteric artery; *SMV,* superior mesenteric vein; *Sp,* spleen; *St,* stomach. *Thick broken line,* retroperitoneal fascia; *thin broken line,* Gerota's fascia; *Solid line,* lateroconal fascia.

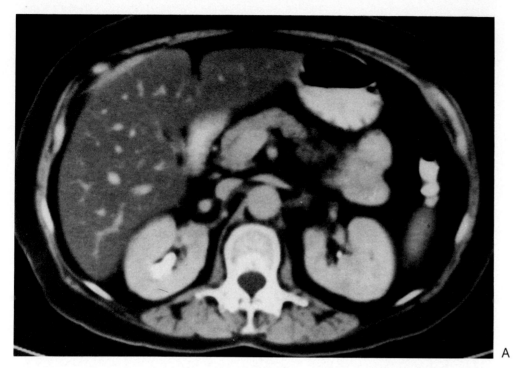

A

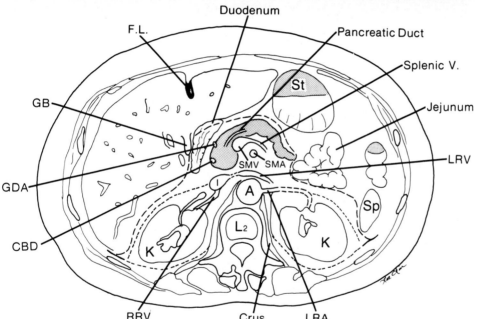

B

Figure 10.19. **A** and **B.** *A,* aorta; *CBD,* common bile duct; *F.L.,* falciform ligament; *GB,* gallbladder; *GDA,* gastroduodenal artery; *I,* inferior vena cava; *K,*
kidney; *LRA,* left renal artery; *LRV,* left renal vein; *RRV,* right renal vein; *SMA,*
superior mesenteric artery; *SMV,* superior mesenteric vein; *Sp,* spleen; *St,*
stomach. *Thick broken line,* retroperitoneal fascia; *thin broken line,* Gerota's
fascia; *solid line,* lateroconal fascia.

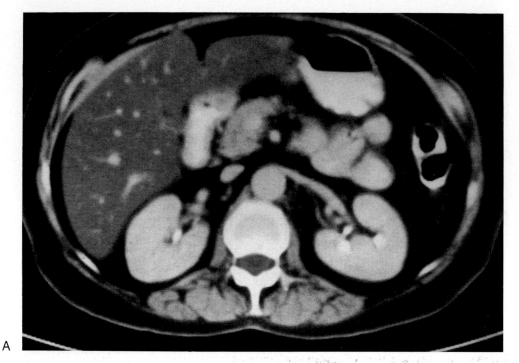

A

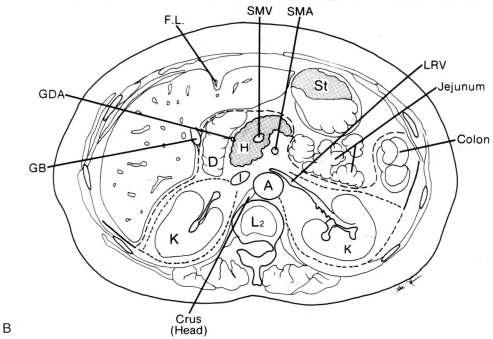

B

Figure 10.20. A and **B.** *A*, aorta; *D*, duodenum (second portion); *F.L.*, falciform ligament; *GB*, gallbladder; *GDA*, gastroduodenal artery; *H*, pancreatic head; *I*, inferior vena cava; *K*, kidney; *LRV*, left renal vein; *SMA*, superior mesenteric artery; *SMV*, superior mesenteric vein; *St*, stomach. *Thick broken line*, retroperitoneal fascia; *think broken line*, Gerota's fascia; *solid line*, lateroconal fascia.

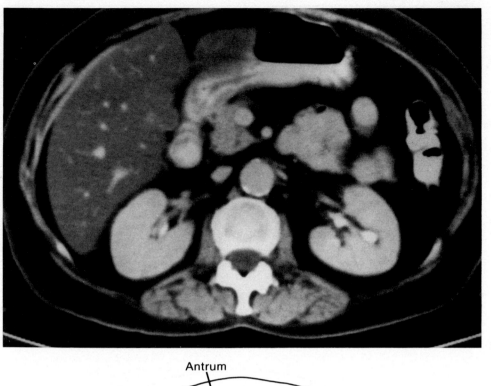

A

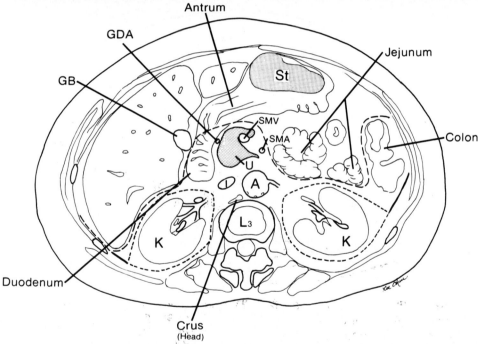

B

Figure 10.21. A and **B.** *A,* aorta; *GB,* gallbladder; *GDA,* gastroduodenal artery; *I,* inferior vena cava; *K,* kidney; *SMA,* superior mesenteric artery; *SMV,* superior mesenteric vein; *St,* stomach; *U,* uncinate process of pancreas. *Thick broken line,* retroperitoneal fascia; *thin broken line,* Gerota's fascia; *solid line,* lateroconal fascia.

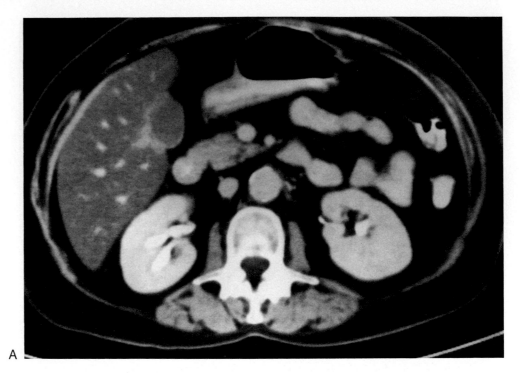

A

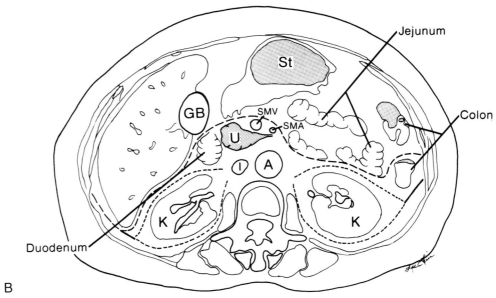

B

Figure 10.22. A and **B.** *A,* aorta; *GB,* gallbladder; *I,* inferior vena cava; *K,* kidney; *SMA,* superior mesenteric artery; *SMV,* superior mesenteric vein; *St,* stomach; *U,* uncinate process of pancreas. *Thick broken line,* retroperitoneal fascia; *thin broken line,* Gerota's fascia; *solid line,* lateroconal fascia.

References and Suggested Readings

1. Balthazar EJ. CT of gastrointestinal tract: Principles and interpretation. *Am J Roetgenol* 1991;156:23–32.
2. Berland LL, VanDyke JA. Decreased splenic enhancement on CT traumatized hypotensive patients. *Radiology* 1985;156:469–471.
3. Burgener FA, Hamlin DJ. Contrast enhancement in abdominal CT: bolus vs infusion. *Am J Roetgenol* 1981;137:351–358.
4. Carr D, Banks LM. Comparison of barium diatrizoate bowel labelling agents in computed tomography. *Br J Radiol* 1985;58:393–394.
5. Chiu LC, Schapiro RL. *Atlas of computed body tomography: normal and abnormal anatomy*. Baltimore: University Park Press, 1980.
6. Cohen WN, Seidelmann FE, Bryan PJ. Use of a tampon to enhance vaginal localization in computed tomography. *Am J Roetgenol* 1977;128:1064–1065.
7. Cranston PE. Colon opacification by oral water-soluble contrast medium administration the night prior to CT examination. *Comput Assist Tomogr* 1982;6:413–415.
8. Foley WD. Dynamic computed tomography with sequential table motion: principles, techniques, and clinical results.
9. Foley WD. Dynamic hepatic CT. *Radiology* 1989;170:617–622.
10. Foley WD, Berland LL, Lawson TL, et al. Contrast enhancement technique for dynamic hepatic computed tomographic scanning. *Radiology* 1983;147:797–803.
11. Haaga JR, Alfidi RJ. *Computed tomography of the whole body*. Vols. I and II. C.V. Mosby: St. Louis, 1983.
12. Hamlin DJ, Burgener FA. Positive and negative contrast agents in CT evaluation of the abdomen and pelvis. *Comput Tomogr* 1981;5:82–90.
13. Hatfield KD, Segal SD, Tait K. Barium sulfate for abdominal computer assisted tomography. *J Comput Assist Tomogr* 1980;4:570.
14. Husband JE, Golding SJ. Computed tomography of the body: when should it be used? *Br Med J* 1982;284:4–7.
15. Kelly J, Raptopoulos V, Davidoff A, et al. The value of non-contrast-enhanced CT in blunt abdominal trauma. *Am J Roetgenol* 1989;152:41–46.
16. Kieffer SA, Heitzman ER. *An atlas of cross-sectional anatomy: computed tomography, ultrasound, radiography, gross anatomy*. Hagerstown, MD: Harper & Row, 1979.
17. Kirkpatrick RH, Wittenberg J, Schaffer DL, et al. Scanning techniques in computed body tomography. *Am J Roetgenol* 1978;130:1069–1075.
18. Koss JC, Arger PH, Coleman BG, et al. CT staging of bladder carcinoma. *Am J Roetgenol* 1981;137:359–362.
19. Lee JKT, Sagel SS, Stanley RJ. *Computed body tomography with MRI correlation*. New York: Raven Press, 1989.
20. Love L, Churchill R, Reynes C, et al. *Use of bolus contrast in computed tomography*. Maywood, IL: Loyola University Medical Center/Foster G. McGaw Hospital, 1981.
21. Marn CS, Francis IR. CT of portal venous occlusion. *Am J Roetgenol* 1992;159:717–726.
22. Megibow AJ, Balthazar EJ, Cho KC, et al. Bowel obstruction: evaluation with CT. *Radiology* 1991;180:313–318.
23. Mintz MC, Seltzer SE. Oral administration of contrast medium for rectal opacification in pelvic computed tomography. *Comput Tomogr* 1984;8:73–74.
24. Mitchell DG, Bjorgvinsson E, terMeulen D, et al. Gastrografin versus dilute barium for colonic CT examinations: a blind randomized study. *J Comput Assist Tomogr* 1985;9:451–453.
25. Moss H, Gamsu G, Genant HK. *Computed tomography of the body*. Philadelphia: W.B. Saunders, 1983.
26. Nakata H, Nakayama T, Kimoto T, et al. Dynamic computed tomography of the pancreas. *J Comput Assist Tomogr* 1982;6:646–649.
27. Nelson RC, Chezmar JL, Peterson JE, et al. Contrast-enhanced CT of the liver and spleen: comparison of ionic and nonionic contrast agents. *Am J Roetgenol* 1989;153:973–976.
28. Neufeld CL. Computed tomography of the abdomen—clinical applications. *AOA* 1981;81:199–206.
29. Rossi P, Baert A, Marchal W, et al. Multiple bolus technique vs single bolus or infusion of contrast medium to obtain prolonged contrast enhancement of the pancrease. *Radiology* 1982;144:929–931.
30. Rossi P, Baert A, Passarielo R, et al. CT of functioning tumors of the pancreas. *Am J Roentgenol* 1985;144:57–60.
31. Rubenstein WA, Auh YH, Zirinsky K, et al. Posterior peritoneal recesses: assessment using CT. *Radiology* 1985;156:461–468.

32. Seidelmann FE, Temes SP, Cohen WN, et al. Computed tomography of gas-filled bladder. *Urology* 1977;9:337–344.

33. Sones PJ. Computed tomography of the retroperitoneum. *Appl Radiol* 1980;9:40–50.

34. Stork J. Intraperitoneal contrast agents for computed tomography. *Am J Roetgenol* 1985;145:300.

35. Takahashi S. *Illustrated computer tomography: a practical guide to CT interpretations.* New York: Springer Verlag, 1983.

36. Tisnado J, Amendola MA, Walsh JW, et al. Computed tomography of the perineum. *Am J Roetgenol* 1981;136:475–481.

37. Wechsler RJ, Nino-Murcia M. Computed tomography of iliopsoas muscle tumors. *Comput Radiol* 1984;8:229–235.

38. Wechsler RJ, Schiling JF. Review CT of the gluteal region. *Am J Roetgenol* 1985;144:185–190.

39. Wolfman NT, Bechtold RE, Scharling ES, et al. Blunt upper abdominal trauma: evaluation by CT. *Am J Roetgenol* 1992;158:493–501.

40. Young SW, Noon MA, Menahem N, et al. Dynamic computed tomography body scanning. *J Comput Assist Tomogr* 1980;4:168–173.

41. Zeman RK, Clements LA, Silverman PM, et al. CT of the liver: a survey of prevailing methods for administration of contrast material. *Am J Roetgenol* 1988;150:107–109.

Male and Female Pelvis: Normal Anatomy

Normal Anatomy of the Male Pelvis

The following series of male (Figs. 11.1 through 11.9) and female (Figs. 11.10 through 11.19) pelvis images were obtained at 95 mA, exposure time of 3.4 sec, 398° scan angle, and a couch index and slice thickness of 10 mm. Intravenous contrast enhancement was attained by a bolus/drip method.

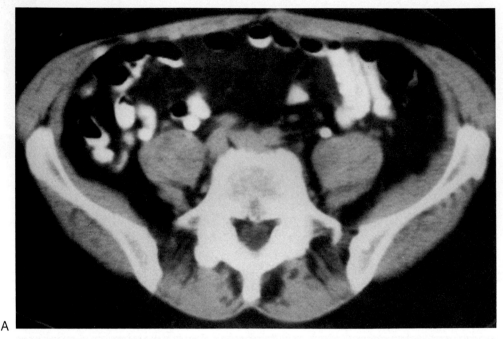

A

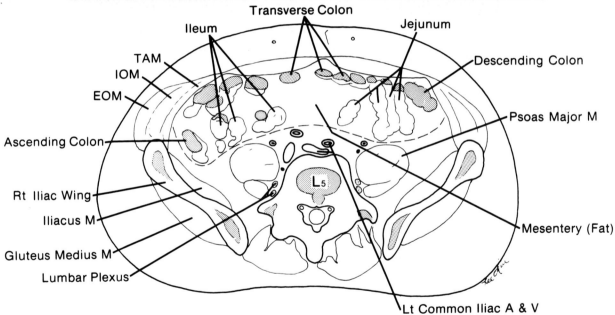

B

Figure 11.1. A and **B.** In this section, the common iliac arteries and veins have become somewhat lateral in position and are just medial to the psoas muscle. The lumbar plexus, which is formed by the union of lumbar nerves, is lateral to the L₅ vertebral body. *EOM,* external oblique muscle; *IOM,* internal oblique muscle; *TAM,* transverse abdominal muscle. *Broken line,* retroperitoneal fascia.

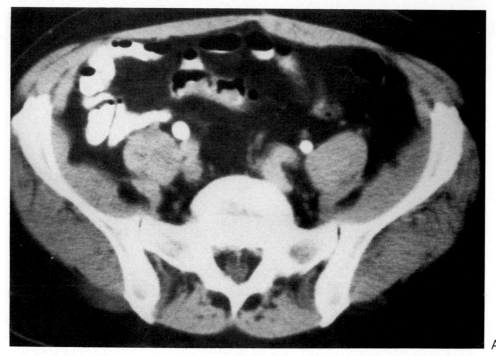

A

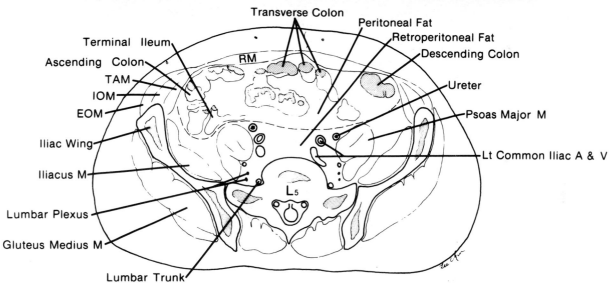

Transverse Colon

Peritoneal Fat

Retroperitoneal Fat

Terminal Ileum

Ascending Colon

RM

Descending Colon

TAM

IOM

EOM

Ureter

Iliac Wing

Psoas Major M

Iliacus M

Lt Common Iliac A & V

Lumbar Plexus

L₅

Gluteus Medius M

Lumbar Trunk

B

Figure 11.2. A and **B.** Scan taken 2 cm distal to the aortic bifurcation. The common iliac arteries are anterior in position to the common iliac veins. The lumbar plexus, which is between the psoas muscle and the L_5 vertebral body, is a network of lumbar nerves. *EOM,* external oblique muscle; *IOM,* internal oblique muscle; *RM,* rectus muscle; *TAM,* transverse abdominal muscle. *Broken line,* retroperitoneal fascia.

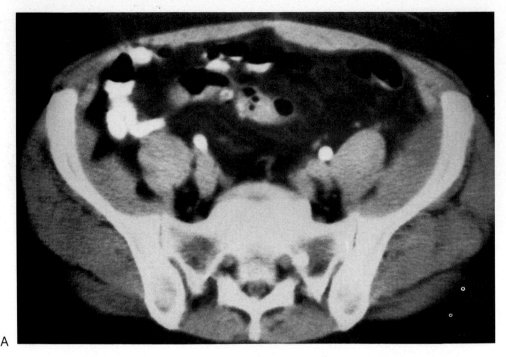

A

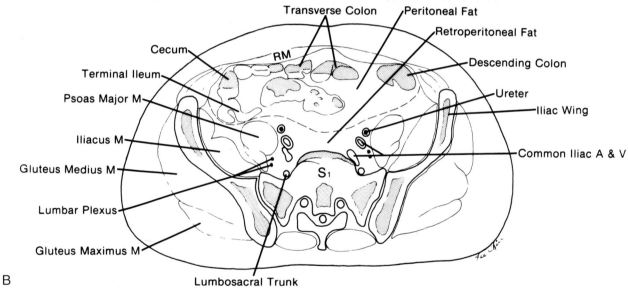

B

Figure 11.3. A and **B.** Section taken at S$_1$. The psoas and iliacus muscles are barely separated by fat. Note the excellent visualization of the ureters, which are anterior to the common iliac arteries and veins. *RM,* rectus muscle. *Broken line,* retroperitoneal fascia.

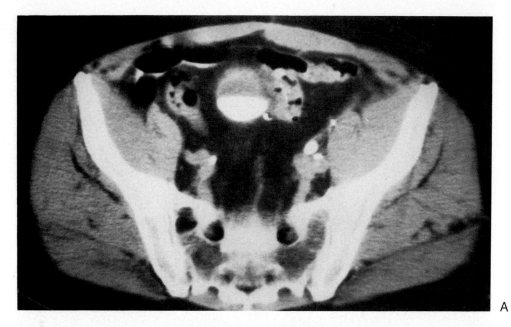

A

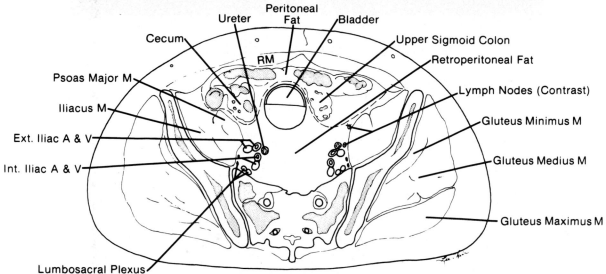

B

Figure 11.4. A and **B.** Section ICM caudal to the common iliac artery and vein bifurcation. The external iliac artery and vein are anterior to the internal artery and vein. Note that there is contrast in the lymph nodes from a previous lymphangiogram. The psoas major muscle has now come in contact with the iliacus muscle and they will form the iliopsoas muscle. *ICM*, 1 cm; *RM*, rectus muscle. *Broken line*, retroperitoneal fascia.

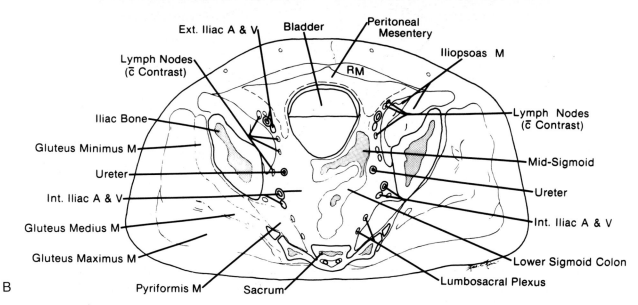

Figure 11.5. A and **B.** The distance between the external and internal arteries and veins has become significantly increased. The external iliac artery and vein now are anterolateral to the iliopsoas muscle. Directly anterior to the pyriformis muscle are the internal iliac artery and vein. *RM,* rectus muscle. *Broken line,* retroperitoneal fascia.

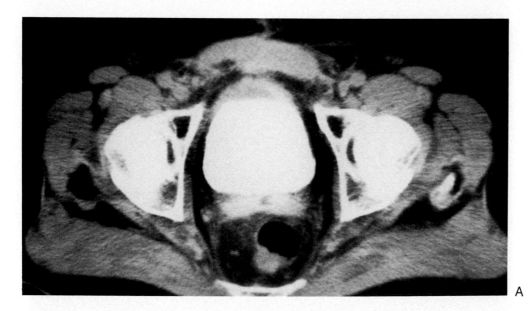

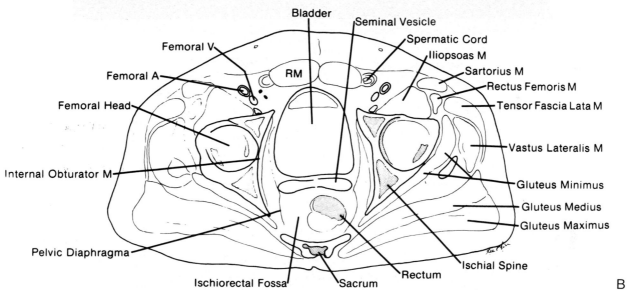

Figure 11.6. A and **B.** Section at the level of the femoral heads. The paired, oval seminal vesicles are seen posterior of the bladder. Those muscles (sartorius, rectus femoris, tensor fascia lata, and vastus lateralis) that allow action of the leg and thigh are seen. *RM,* rectus muscle.

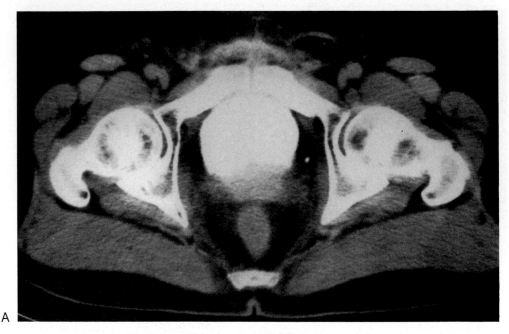

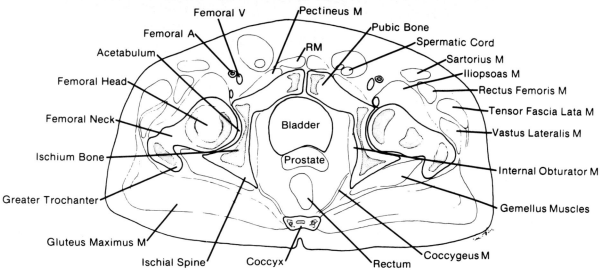

Figure 11.7. A and **B.** Scan taken at the level of the symphysis pubis. The top portion of the prostate can be seen. The spermatic cords are visualized anterior to the pectineus muscle. The pectineus muscle aids in movement of the thigh. *RM,* rectus muscle.

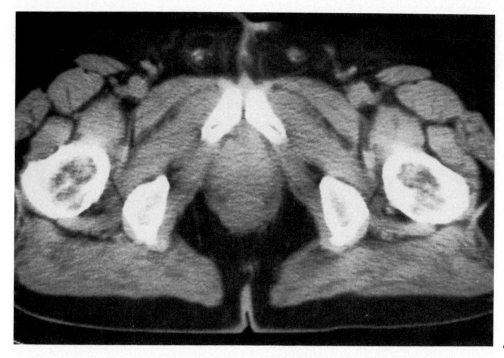

A

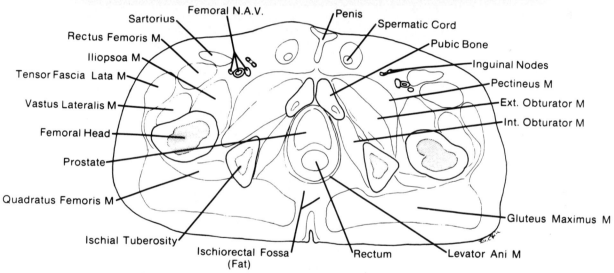

B

Figure 11.8. A and **B.** Section through the lower portion of the symphysis pubis. Note that the prostate lies directly posterior of the symphysis pubis. The spermatic cords are easily seen on either side of the top portion of the penis. Easily distinguishable in this patient by fat planes are the internal and external obturator muscles, which allow lateral rotation of the thigh.

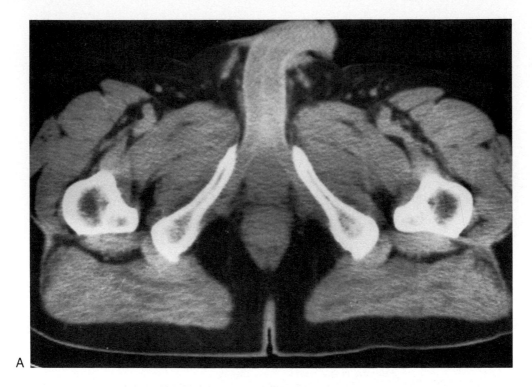

A

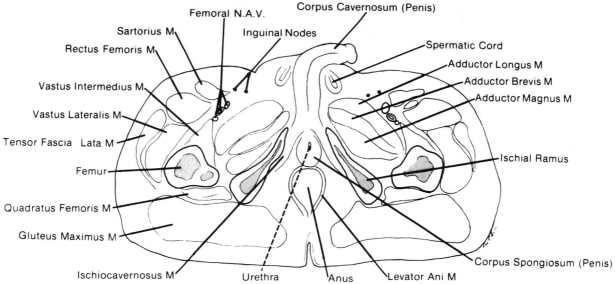

B

Figure 11.9. A and **B.** Scan at the ischial ramus shows the penile portion of the urethra. The three adductor muscles, which serve the function of adduction of the thigh, are seen.

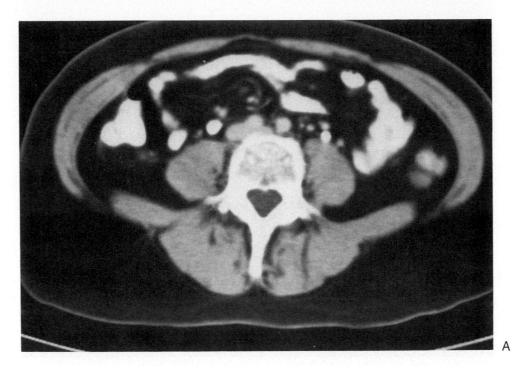

A

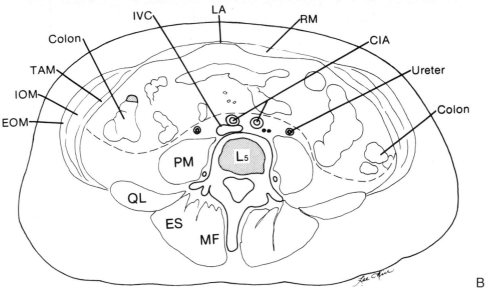

B

Figure 11.10. A and **B.** Scan taken 2 cm below the aortic bifurcation. *CIA,* common iliac artery; *EOM,* external oblique muscle; *ES,* erector spinal muscle; *IOM,* internal oblique muscle; *IVC,* inferior vena cava; *LA,* linea alba; *MF,* multifidus muscle; *PM,* psoas muscle; *QL,* quadratus lumborum muscle; *RM,* rectus muscle; *TAM,* transverse abdominal muscle. *Broken line,* retroperitoneal fascia.

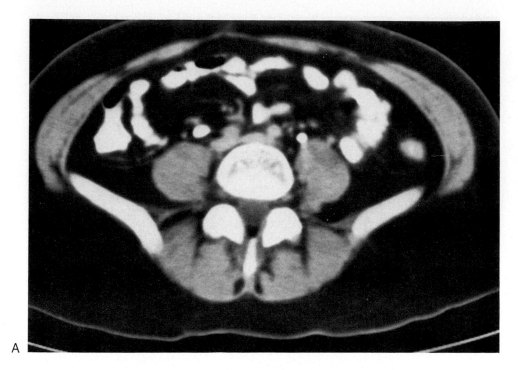

A

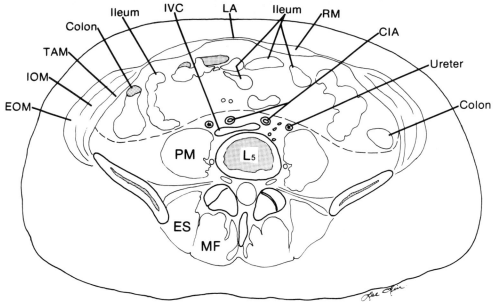

B

Figure 11.11. **A** and **B.** Section at the iliac crest. *CIA*, common iliac artery; *ES*, erector spinal muscle; *EOM*, external oblique muscle; *IOM*, internal oblique muscle; *IVC*, inferior vena cava; *LA*, linea alba; *MF*, multifidus muscle; *PM*, psoas muscle; *RM*, rectus muscle; *TAM*, transverse abdominal muscle. *Broken line*, retroperitoneal fascia.

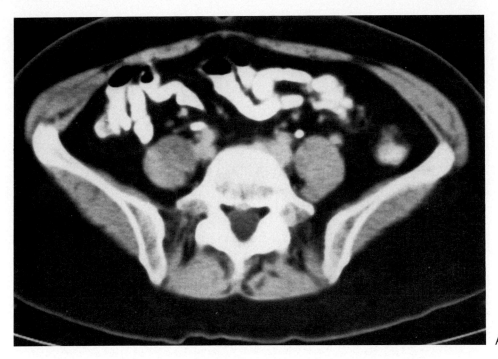

A

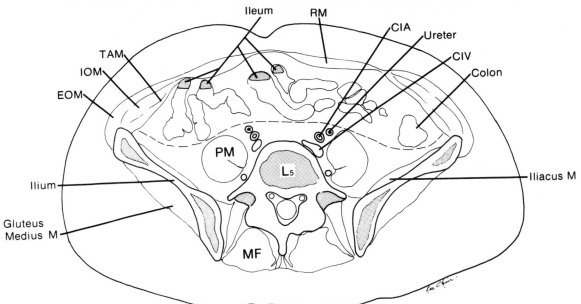

B

Figure 11.12. A and **B.** Scan taken approximately 2 cm distal to the bifurcation of the inferior vena cava. *CIA,* common iliac artery; *CIV,* common iliac vein; *EOM,* external oblique muscle; *IOM,* internal oblique muscle; *MF,* multifidus muscle; *PM,* psoas muscle; *RM,* rectus muscle; *TAM,* transverse abdominal muscle. *Broken line,* retroperitoneal fascia.

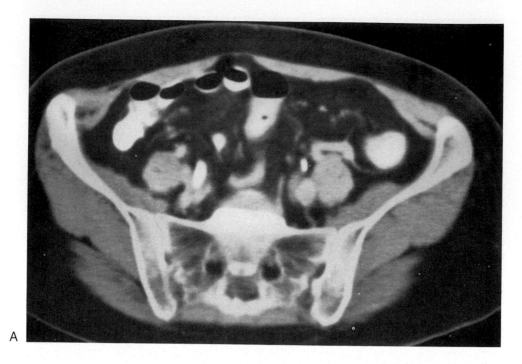

A

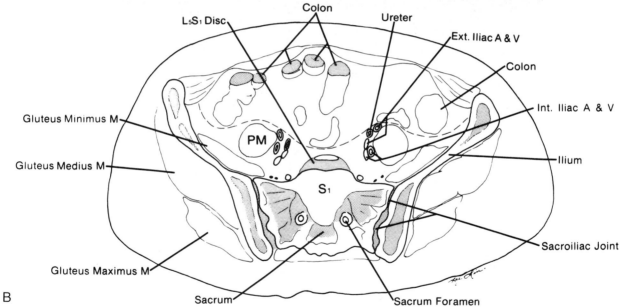

B

Figure 11.13. A and **B.** Scan at the level of L₅–S₁ intervertebral disc. *PM*, psoas muscle. *Broken line*, retroperitoneal fascia.

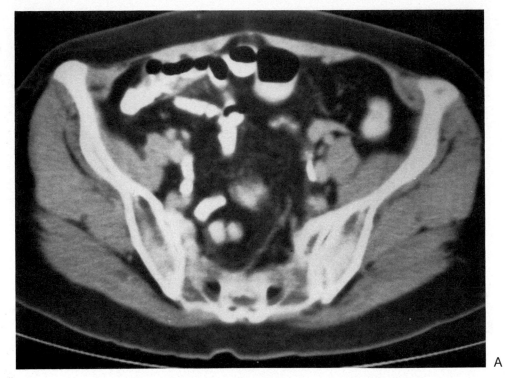

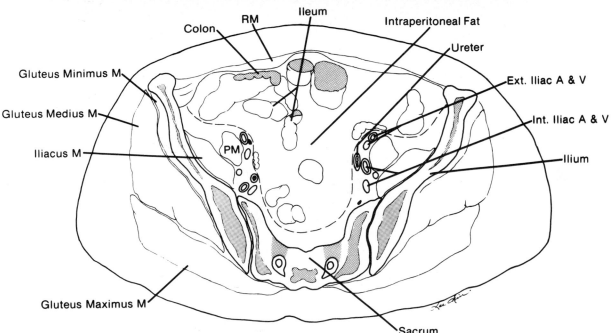

Figure 11.14. A and **B.** At this level, the three gluteal muscles are distinctively seen because of the excellent fat planes. *PM,* psoas muscle; *RM,* rectus muscle. *Broken line,* retroperitoneal fascia.

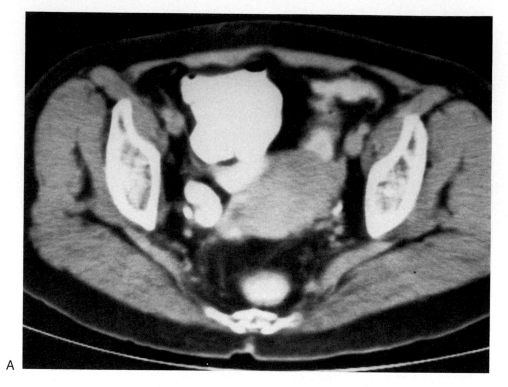

A

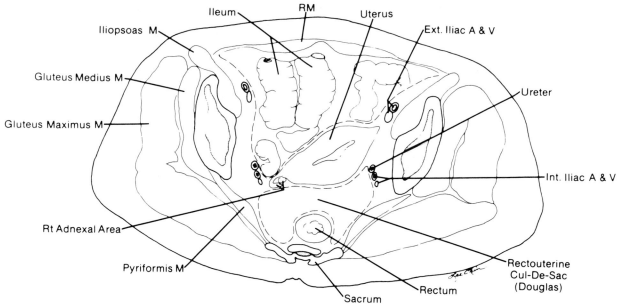

B

Iliopsoas M

Gluteus Medius M

Gluteus Maximus M

Rt Adnexal Area

Pyriformis M

Ileum

RM

Uterus

Ext. Iliac A & V

Ureter

Int. Iliac A & V

Rectouterine
Cul-De-Sac
(Douglas)

Rectum

Sacrum

Figure 11.15. A and **B.** Scan at the level of the uterus. The adnexal area on the right is well seen. The uterine adnexa are composed of accessory structures of the uterus such as the ovaries and uterine tubes. *RM*, rectus muscle. *Broken line*, retroperitoneal fascia.

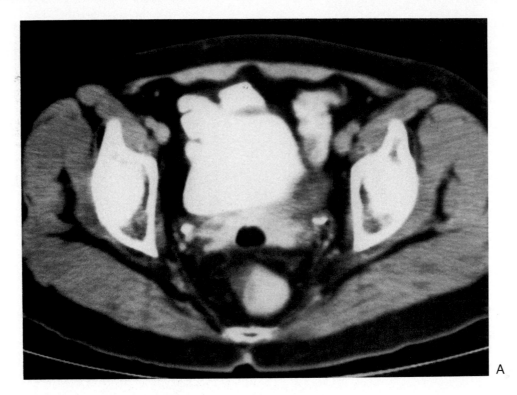

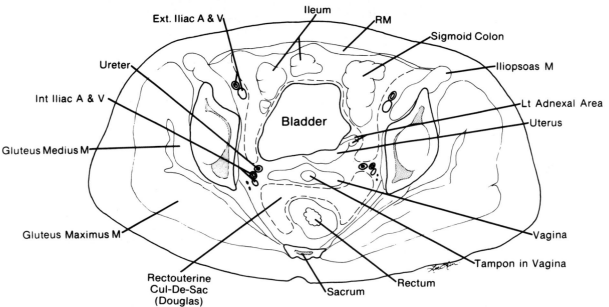

Figure 11.16. A and **B.** Scan taken at the level of the femoral heads shows good definition of the vagina due to insertion of a tampon. *RM*, rectus muscle. *Broken line*, retroperitoneal fascia.

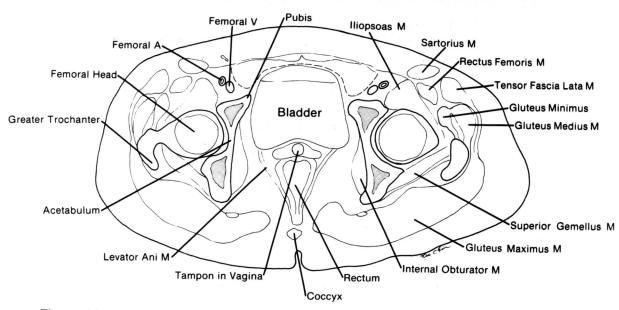

Figure 11.17. A and **B.** In this cross-section at the level of the acetabulum, the levator ani muscle is seen along the lateral margin of the rectum. The levator ani muscle assists in support of the pelvic viscera. *Broken line,* retroperitoneal fascia.

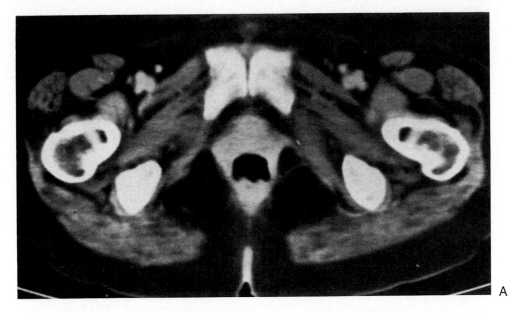

A

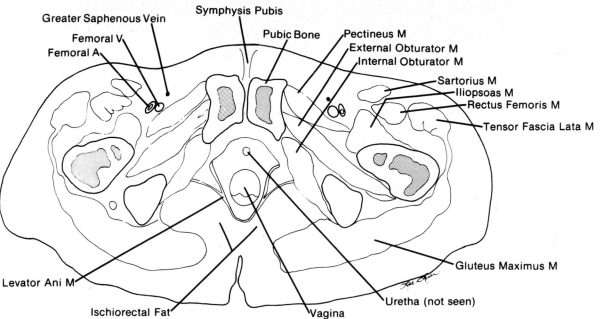

B

Figure 11.18. A and **B.** Scan at the symphysis pubis. There is easy visualization of the femoral artery and vein due to enhancement. Note the greater saphenous vein, which is also well seen medial to the femoral vein.

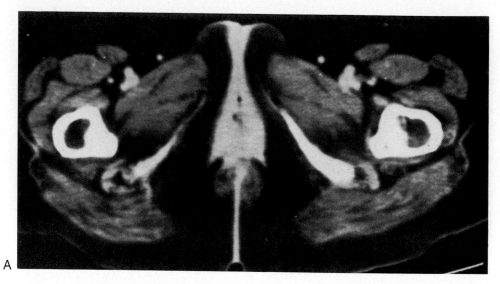

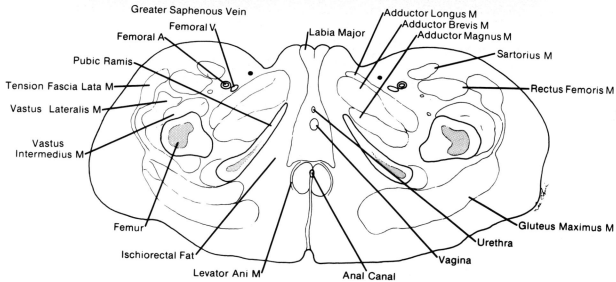

Figure 11.19. A and **B.** Scan 3 cm below the symphysis pubis shows the urethra anterior to the vagina. Seen as the most anterior structure are the labia major. The labia major are two rounded folds of fatty tissue, which are part of the vulva.

Spine

Positioning

For viewing the spine, the patient is in the supine position with hands above the head. Flexing the hips and knees helps reduce the lordotic lumbar curve when scanning the lumbar spine.

Occasionally the patient is not able to tolerate the supine position and in such cases the prone position may have to be used. When the prone position is necessary, it must be remembered to change the patient's orientation on the scanning protocol.

The specific area of the spine to be examined determines whether a lateral or a posterior–anterior (PA) localizer is used for positioning. A lateral localizer is ideal for positioning the lumbar spine because of the ease of counting the vertebral bodies from the sacrum. A PA localizer should be used for positioning the thoracic spine, as anatomical localization is easier owing to visibility of the ribs.

Technique

Two methods of scanning are routinely used to investigate the spine. One method is to scan with gantry angulation parallel to the intervertebral disc space. the other is to scan the spine without gantry angulation.

For both methods, a slice thickness and couch index of 4–5 mm are routinely used because they give good visualization of both the spine and the surrounding structures. Smaller or larger increments are used occasionally for evaluation of small or gross pathology. If optimal coronal and sagittal reformations are needed, an overlap in slice thickness and couch index should be used. An example of this would be a 4-mm thickness and 3-mm couch index.

With Angulation

Examining the spine with slices parallel to the intervertebral disc space is used in cases where herniated discs are suspected. This method, which is popular for examinations of the lumbar spine, is performed in the following manner: a lateral localizer is taken, and the gantry tilt required for the involved discs is measured with the cursor. Angles are changed at the middle of the vertebral body preceding the involved intervertebral disc. This technique allows viewing of the intervertebral disc and spinal canal without distortion. One disadvantage of this technique is that coronal, sagittal, and oblique reformations are degraded by the angle changes.

Without Angulation

This method of examining the spine without angulation is ideal in studies where spinal cord lesions are suspected. Often, accurate coronal, sagittal, and oblique reformations are needed to define a lesion's extension and relationship to other structures. Because there is no change in orientation of the scanning plane in this technique, reformations are accurate.

Scanning without angulation is also used for evaluation of herniated discs. After the area of interest is scanned, sections are imaged parallel to the intervertebral disc space.

Contrast Enhancement

METRIZAMIDE CT

Intrathecal metrizamide CT allows a more extensive look at spinal pathology. In patients who are obese or have larger shoulders, fluoroscopic myelography often cannot provide adequate visualization of the low cervical or high thoracic area. In addition, although fluoroscopic myelography can show spinal blocks or compression, it often cannot accurately determine the etiology of such conditions. In these situations, CT can be very beneficial because of its ability to provide cross-sectional images as well as coronal, sagittal, and oblique reformations all of which help in determining if the cord compression or displacement is induced by bone or soft tissue masses.

A water-soluble intrathecal contrast solvent (e.g., metrizamide), which mixes well with cerebrospinal fluid (CSF) and has a low viscosity, gives good visualization of the spinal cord and nerve roots after introduction by injection into the subarachnoid space.

Before examinations, particularly of the lumbar spine, patients should be rolled over several times to ensure mixing of the metrizamide and CSF. Metrizamide often layers out, particularly in the lumbar portion of the subarachnoid space. When scanning patients after instillation of metrizamide, it is of paramount importance to keep the head elevated to prevent draining of metrizamide into the head, which can cause headaches, nausea, vomiting, and seizures.

INTRAVENOUS CONTRAST MEDIA

Intravenous (IV) contrast is not used frequently to examine the spine, especially the lumbar spine, because of the inherent contrast produced by epidural fat, nerve roots, and ligamentum flavum. When used, IV contrast enhances the dura by way of the dural veins. IV contrast is often used on postoperative patients who are suspected of having a ruptured disc. By using contrast, a distinction may be made between fibrotic scarring and a ruptured disc due to enhancement of the scarring (20).

SOFT TISSUE AND BONE IMAGING

The spine should be viewed at two different window widths (WW) and window levels (WL) so both soft tissue and bone can be accurately examined. When adjusting the WW and WL for examining soft tissue, settings are used in which there is fine visualization of spinal cord, nerve roots, intervertebral discs, and ligamentum flavum. To examine bony structure, the WW and WL are adjusted so that there is sharp definition of bony contour, e.g., distinct outline of the articular joint.

If scanning is done on patients injected with water-soluble intrathecal contrast 2 hours or less after injection, bone imaging settings are needed. The high density of intrathecal contrast makes visualization of paraspinal structures difficult.

NORMAL ANATOMY OF THE SPINE

The following series of spinal images (Figs. 12.1 through 12.12) were performed by angulating the gantry parallel to the intervertebral disc space. A setting of 65 mA, an exposure time of 9.3 sec, and a 360° scan angle were used; the slice thickness and couch index were 4 mm.

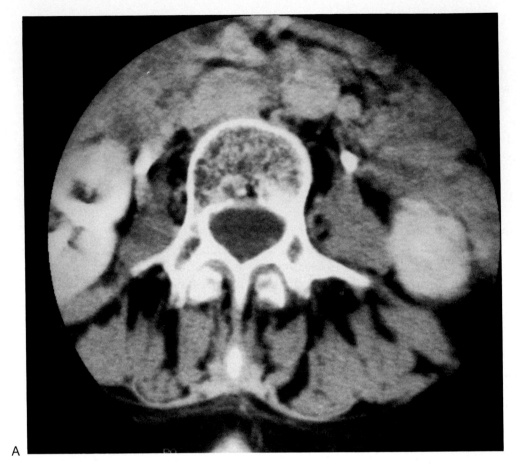

A

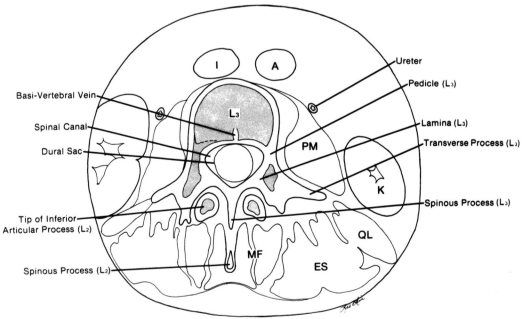

B

Figure 12.1. A and **B.** CT scan at the middle of L₃. The basivertebral vein is noted directly anterior to the thecal sac. It is this vein that drains the vertebral bodies. Easily seen are the right kidney and ureteres due to intravenous contrast. *A,* aorta; *ES,* erector spinal muscle; *I,* inferior vena cava; *K,* kidney; *MF,* multifidus muscle; *PM,* psoas muscle; *QL,* quadratus lumborum muscle.

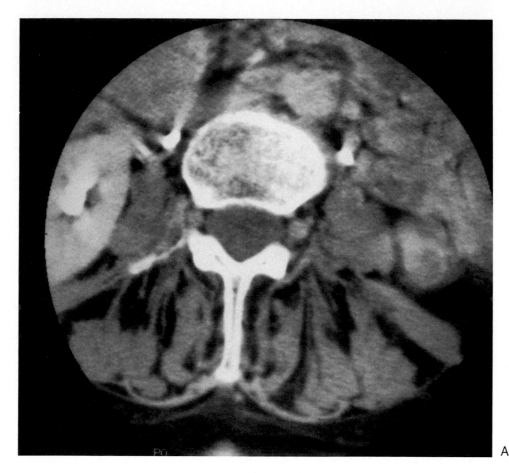

A

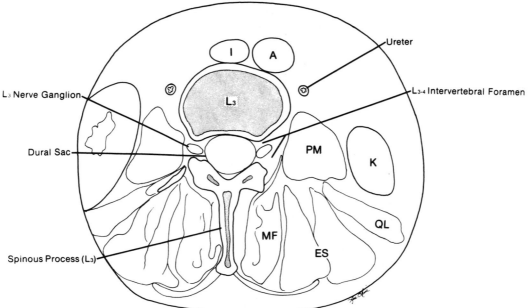

B

Figure 12.2. A and **B.** CT scan at L₃ inferior to the pedicles. The L₃ nerve ganglion are seen exiting through the L₃–L₄ intervertebral foramen. Note the density of the dural sac as compared to the L₃ nerve ganglion. *A,* aorta; *ES,* erector spinal muscle; *I,* inferior vena cava; *K,* kidney; *MF,* multifidus muscle; *PM,* psoas muscle; *QL,* quadratus lumborum muscle.

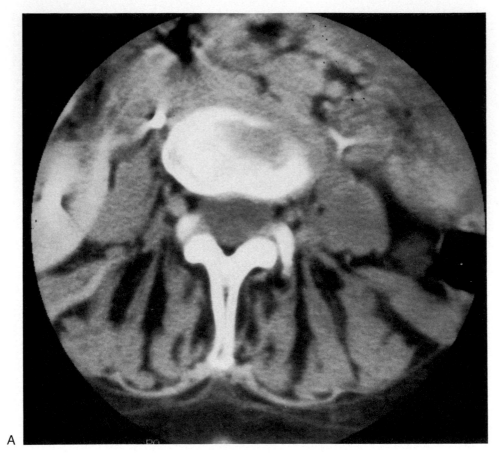

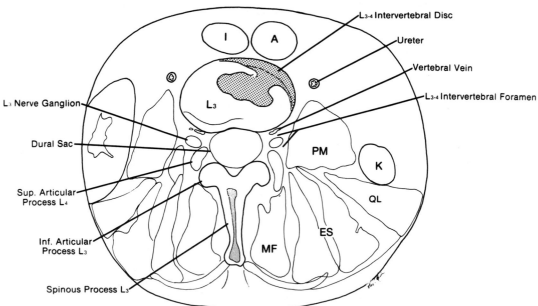

Figure 12.3. A and **B.** Cross-section through the lower part of the L₃–L₄ intervertebral foraman. *A*, aorta; *ES*, erector spinal muscle; *I*, inferior vena cava; *K*, kidney; *MF*, multifidus muscle; *PM*, psoas muscle; *QL*, quadratus lumborum muscle.

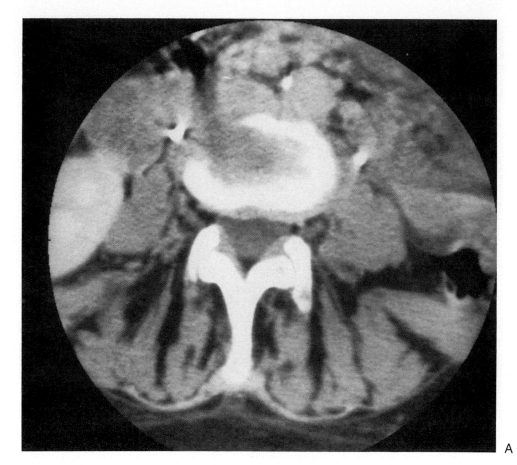

A

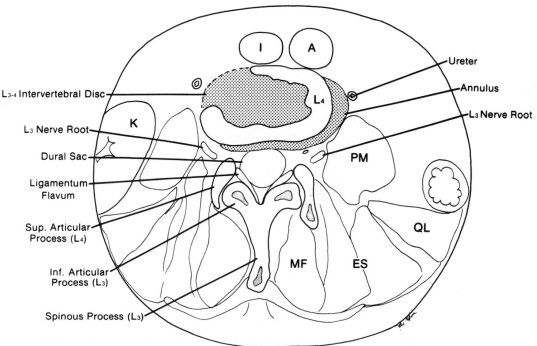

L₃₋₄ Intervertebral Disc

L₃ Nerve Root

Dural Sac

Ligamentum Flavum

Sup. Articular Process (L₄)

Inf. Articular Process (L₃)

Spinous Process (L₃)

Ureter

Annulus

L₃ Nerve Root

I   A

K

L₄

PM

QL

MF   ES

B

Figure 12.4. A and **B.** CT scan at the L₃–L₄ intervertebral disc. The density of this disc is higher than the adjacent dural sac. At this level the superior articular process of the inferior vertebra *(L₄)* and inferior articular process of the superior vertebra *(L₃)* are seen forming the apophyseal (facet) joint. *A,* aorta; *ES,* erector spinal muscle; *I,* inferior vena cava; *K,* kidney, *MF,* multifidus muscle; *PM,* psoas muscle; *QL,* quadratus lumborum muscle.

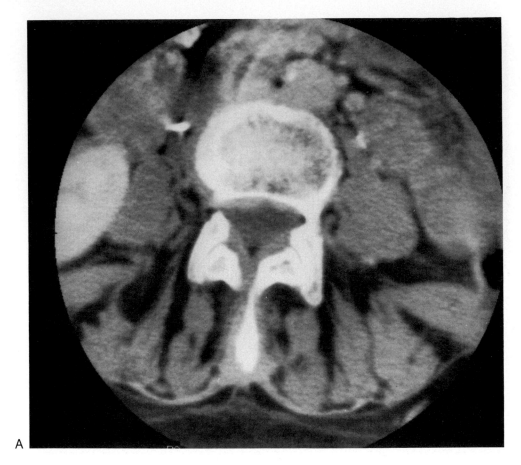

A

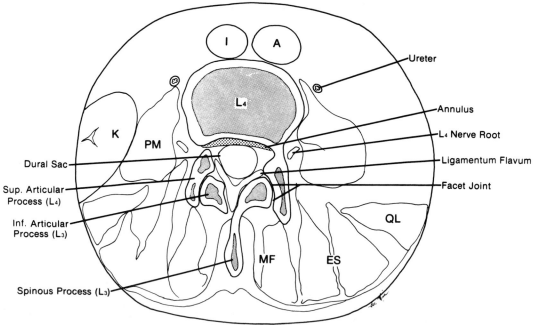

B

Figure 12.5. A and **B.** Scan taken at the top of L$_4$ vertebral body. There is excellent demonstration of the ligamentum flavum in this slice. The outer portion of the disc (annulus) is seen outlining the anterior border of the thecal sac. *A,* aorta; *ES,* erector spinal muscle; *I,* inferior vena cava; *K,* kidney; *MF,* multifidus muscle; *PM,* psoas muscle; *QL,* quadratus lumborum muscle.

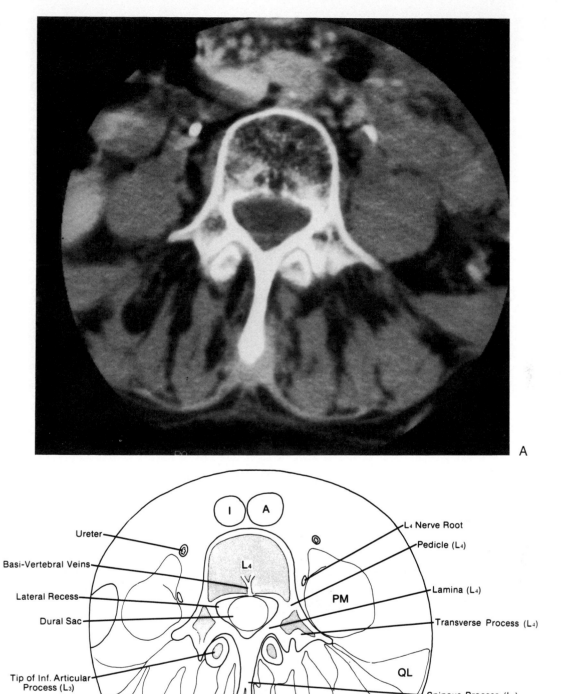

Figure 12.6. A and **B.** CT scan of the mid-L₄ vertebral body. The lamina and pedicles form the vertebral arch. The tip of the inferior articular process of L₃ is seen. Again note the basi-vertebral vein. *A,* aorta; *ES,* erector spinal muscle; *I,* inferior vena cava; *MF,* multifidus muscle; *PM,* psoas muscle; *QL,* quadratus lumborum muscle.

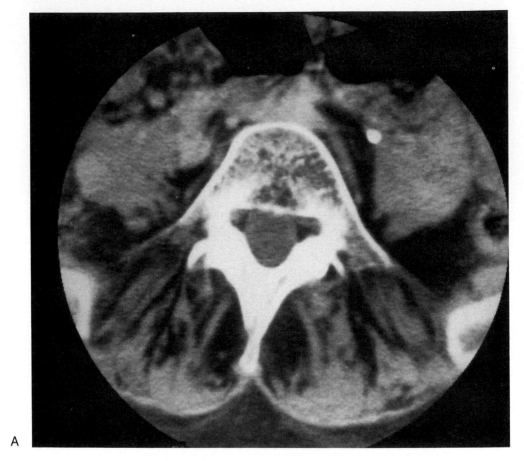

A

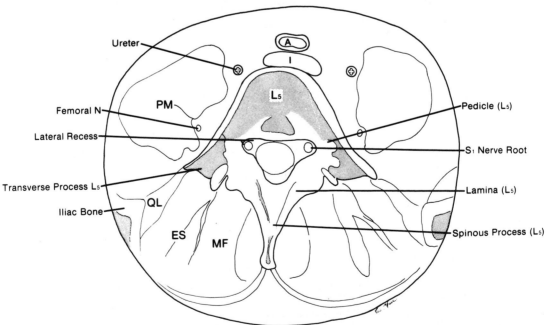

B

Figure 12.7. A and **B.** CT scan of the mid-L$_5$ vertebral body. The S$_1$ nerve roots are situated in the lateral recesses. The lateral recess is formed anteriorly by the posterior vertebral body, laterally by the pedicle, and posteriorly by the lamina. *A,* aorta; *ES,* erector spinal muscle; *I,* inferior vena cava; *MF,* multifidus muscle; *PM,* psoas muscle; *QL,* quadratus lumborum muscle.

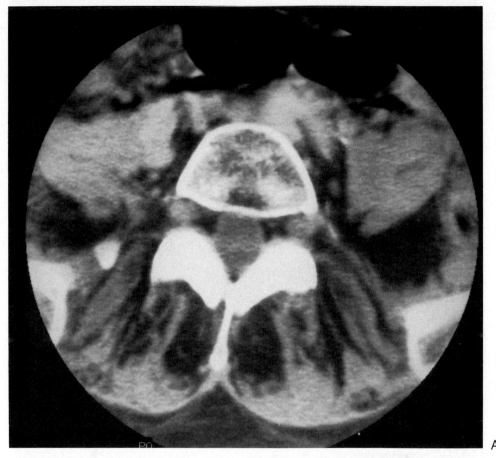

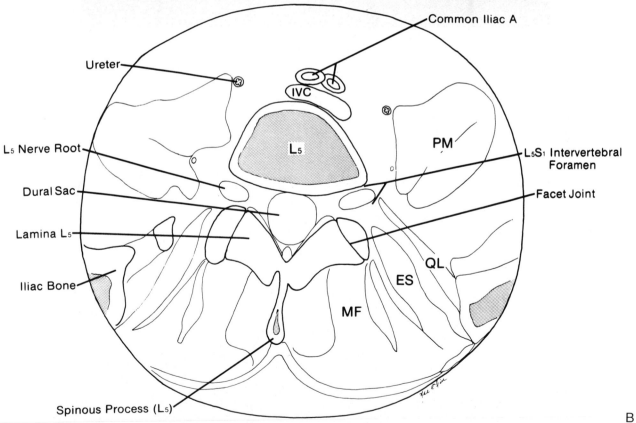

Figure 12.8. A and **B.** Scan at the level of the L_5–S_1 intervertebral foramen. The L_5 nerve roots and dural sac are easily seen owing to epidural fat, which is surrounding the dural sac. The aorta has bifurcated into the right and left common iliac arteries. *ES,* erector spinal muscle; *IVC,* inferior vena cava; *MF,* multifidus muscle; *PM,* psoas muscle; *QL,* quadratus lumborum muscle.

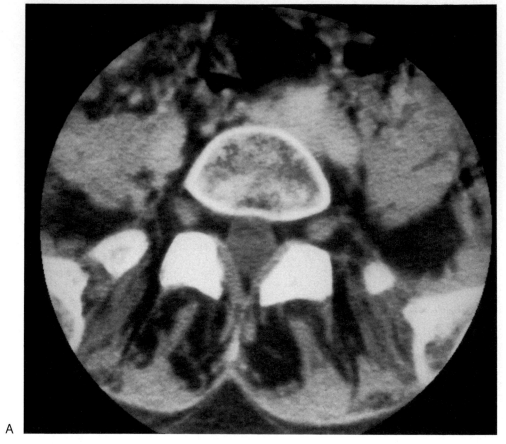

A

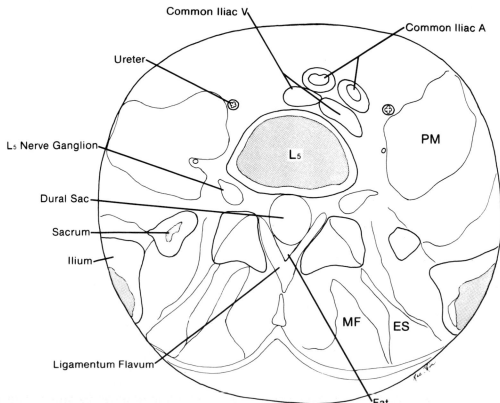

B

Figure 12.9. A and **B.** CT scan 8 mm inferior to the L₅ pedicles shows the L₅ nerve ganglion coursing through the intervertebral foramen. The inferior vena cava has bifurcated into the right and left common iliac veins. *ES*, erector spinal muscle; *MF*, multifidus muscle; *PM*, psoas muscle.

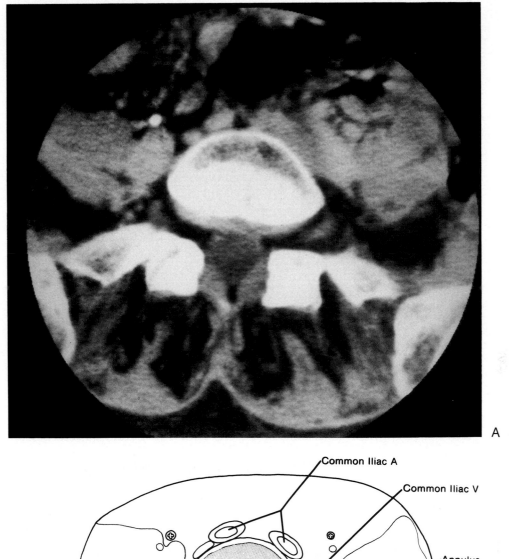

A

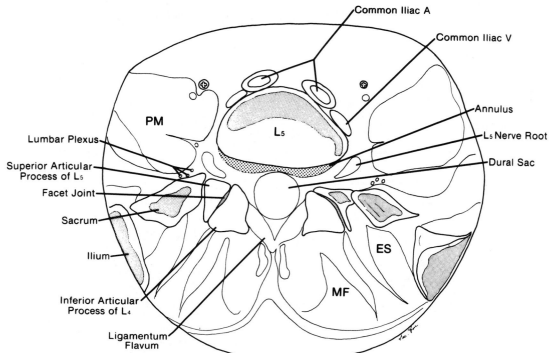

B

Figure 12.10. A and **B.** Cross-section at the bottom of L₅. The superior articular process of L₅ and inferior articular process of L₄ are seen forming the apophyseal (facet) joint. *ES,* erector spinal muscle; *MF,* multifidus muscle; *PM,* psoas muscle.

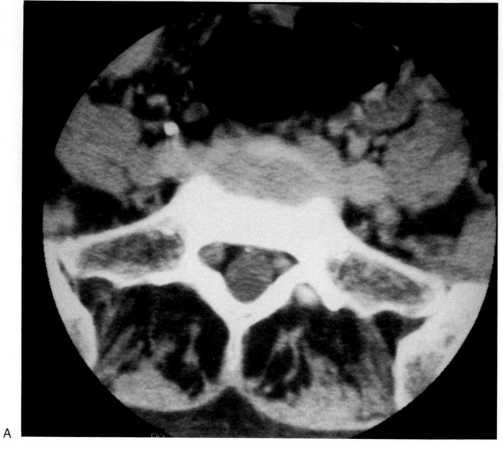

A

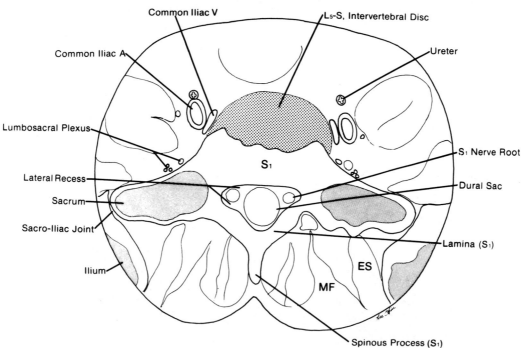

B

Figure 12.11. A and **B.** CT scan at L_5–S_1 intervertebral disc. By scanning parallel to the intervertebral disc, only partial visualization is made of the L_5–S_1 disc. Because of the immense angle of this disc space, the maximum −20° gantry tilt was not enough to obtain a parallel scanning plane. The common iliac arteries and veins are medial to the psoas muscle. *ES*, erector spinal muscle; *MF*, multifidus muscle.

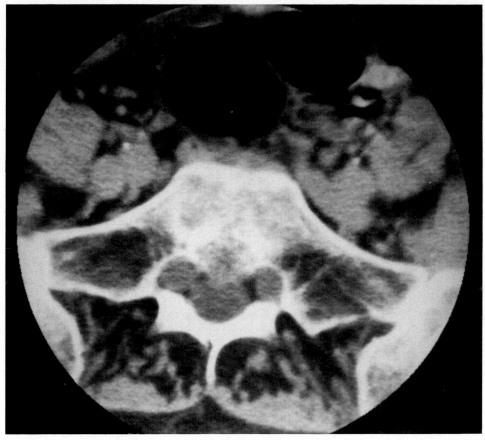

A

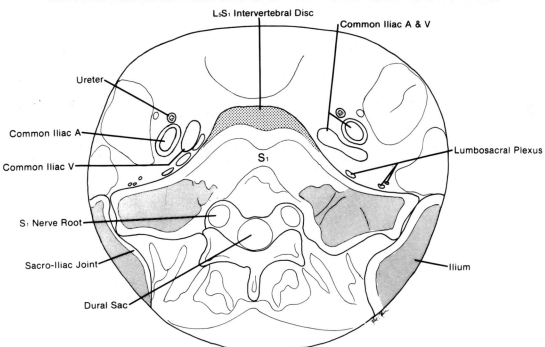

B

Figure 12.12. A and **B.** Scan taken at the superior portion of S₁ gives fine visualization of the S₁ nerve roots and their normal relationship to the dural sac. Note the "mouse ear" image that the S₁ nerve roots give to the dural sac.

References and Suggested Readings

1. Anand AK, Lee BCP. Plain and metrizamide CT of lumbar disk disease: comparison with myelography. *Am J Neuroradiol* 1982;3:567–571.
2. Braun IF, Lin JP, Benjamin MV, et al. Computed tomography of the asymptomatic post-surgical spine: analysis of the physiologic scar. *Am J Roetgenol* 1984;142:149–152.
3. Coin CG, Herman GT, Coin JT. Computed tomography of the spine: techniques and procedures. *Comput Radiol* 1982;6:69–74.
4. Dake MD, Jacobs RP, Margolin FR. Computed tomography of posterior lumbar apophyseal ring fractures. *J Comput Assist Tomogr* 1985;9:730–732.
5. Fing IJ, Garra BS, Zabell A, et al. Computed tomography with metrizamide myelography to define the extent of spinal block due to tumor. *J Comput Assist Tomogr* 1984; 8:1072–1075.
6. Fries JW, Abodeely DA, Vijungco JG, et al. Computed tomography of herniated and extruded nucleus pulposus. *J Comput Assist Tomogr* 1982;6:874–887.
7. Genant HK, Chafetz N, Helms CA. *Computed tomography of the lumbar spine: diagnostic and therapeutic implications for the radiologist, orthopedist, and neurosurgeon.* San Francisco: University of California Printing Department, 1982.
8. Goldberg AL, Soo MSC, Deeb ZL, et al. Degenerative disease of the lumbar spine: role of CT-myelography in the MR era. *Clin Imaging* 1991;15:47–55.
9. Gulati AN, Weinstein R, Studdard E. CT scan of the spine for herniated discs. *Neuroradiology* 1981;22:57–60.
10. Haughton VM. *Computed tomography of the spine.* St. Louis: C.V. Mosby, 1982.
11. Heithoff KB. High-resolution computed tomography of the lumbar spine. *Postgrad Med* 1981;70:193–208.
12. Hirschy JC, Leue WM, Berninger WH, et al. CT of the lumbosacral spine: importance of tomographic planes parallel to vertebral end plate. *Am J Roetgenol* 1981;136:47–52.
13. Kittredge RD. Computed tomographic evaluation of the thoracic prevertebral and paravertebral spaces. *J Comput Tomogr* 1983;7:239–250.
14. Naidich TP, King DG, Moran CJ, et al. Computed tomography of the lumbar thecal sac. *J Comput Assist Tomogr* 1980;4:37–41.
15. Petras AF, Sobel DF, Mani JR, et al. CT myelography in cervical nerve root avulsion. *J Comput Assist Tomogr* 1985;9:275–279.
16. Raskin SP. Demonstration of nerve roots on unenhanced computed tomographic scans. *J Comput Assist Tomogr* 1981;5:281–284.
17. Roub LW, Drayer BP. Spinal computed tomography: limitations and applications. *Am J Roetgenol* 1979;133:267–273.
18. Schnebel B, Kinston S, Watkins R, et al. Comparison of MRI to contrast CT in the diagnosis of spinal stenosis. *Spine* 1989;14:332–337.
19. Stockley I, Getty CJM, Dixon AK, et al. Lumbar lateral canal entrapment: Clinical, radiculographic and computed tomographic findings. *Clin Radiol* 1988;39:144–149.
19. Taylor AJ, Haughton VM, Doust BD. CT imaging of the thoracic spinal cord without intrathecal contrast medium. *J Comput Assist Tomogr* 1980;4:223–224.
20. Teplick JG, Haskin ME. Intravenous contrast-enhanced CT of the postoperative lumbar spine: improved identification of recurrent disk herniation, scar, arachnoiditis, and diskitis. *Am J Roetgenol* 1984;143:845–855.
21. Williams V, Pickus M, Melamde JL. Computed tomography of the lumbar spine. *Appl Radiol* 1983;12:89–99.

13

Spiral CT: A New Alternative

Diane O'Dell, B.S.R.T.

A new breakthrough in CT technology is Spiral (helical) CT. This new and advanced scan technique has become available because of the continuous rotation of both the x-ray tube and the detector in a circle around the patient.

Spiral CT is a continuous data acquisition as the patient travels through the gantry aperture at a constant speed. (See Fig. 13.1). This allows an entire area of interest to be covered in a single breathhold, which eliminates respiratory motion and inconsistencies due to patient breathing. Most patients do not breathhold the same volume of air for each breathhold command. Spiral CT provides us with gap-free slices and eliminates the delay between scans.

Thus, spiral CT has progressed even further than our standard dynamic CT. During a dynamic CT mode, a 1-sec scan is obtained, but then there is time spent on table incrementation and possibly on image reconstruction before a second scan can be acquired. This could lead to an interscan delay of 5–9 sec and also a loss of vascular enhancement. Therefore, spiral CT allows scanning during optimal vessel opacification and has the ability to acquire image data through the area of interest in a matter of seconds. The acquired spiral data can then be reconstructed as often as necessary and at any table position. The data can also be reconstructed with overlapping images resulting in high-quality multiplanar and three-dimensional images.

D. O'Dell: Department of Radiology, University of North Carolina, School of Medicine, Chapel Hill, North Carolina 27599.

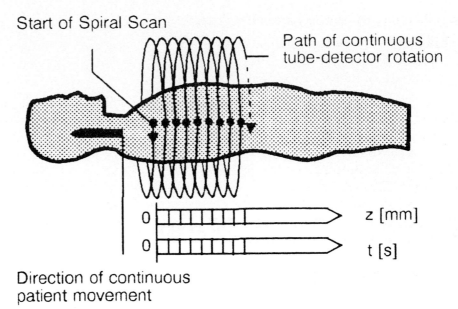

Start of Spiral Scan

Path of continuous tube-detector rotation

z [mm]

t [s]

Direction of continuous patient movement

Figure 13.1. Spiral-shaped scan technique with continuous radiation and simultaneous table movement. (Courtesy of Siemens Medical Systems.)

Technique

The patients are prepped exactly as they would be for a nonspiral exam. If ordered, oral contrast is given 30–45 minutes before starting the examination to ensure good bowel opacification. In most cases, venous access is also obtained for injection of IV contrast material. (A 20-gauge or larger angio-catheter should be placed, preferably in a medially directed antecubital vein.) Due to the shorter scan times, the contrast should be injected at a rate of 2–3 ml/sec by a power injector. Shorter scan times could also lead to a decrease in the total volume of IV contrast that is administered to the patient. This could reduce the risk of renal shutdown and also reduce patient costs. The patients should also be instructed on how to hold their breath during the scan. For spiral scans that require longer scan times, we have found it helpful to hyperventilate the patients immediately before starting the spiral scan. This seems to allow them to hold their breath longer.

Once the range or area of interest to be covered has been programmed, the spiral menu can be pulled up. This menu allows the technologist the ability to set up the scan parameters that will be required for the exam. The following are some examples of the scan parameter choices:

Algorithm	Table speed—should be equal to slice thickness
Slice thickness (collimation)	Table direction
Milliamperage	Feed correction
Time—maximum of 40 seconds	Data storage—yes

The milliamperage and time are determined by the length of the area of interest to be covered and also by the slice thickness at which it is acquired.

The milliamperage settings are often limited to the following times:

1. Maximum of 16 sec using 250 mA
2. Maximum of 32 sec using 210 mA
3. Maximum of 40 sec using 165 mA

Thus, if a large area needs to be covered, a smaller milliamperage is required. Collimation (slice thickness) also directly affects milliampere selection. For example, if the area of interest to be covered is 30 cm in length and you want to cover the area with 10 mm collimation (or a 10-mm slice thickness), you could choose the higher 210-mA level and cover the area in less than 32 seconds (one scan rotation per second). But, if the same area of interest needs to be covered with an 8-mm slice thickness, you would need more than 32 seconds to cover a 30-cm area. Therefore, your milliamperage would have to be decreased to 165 mA in order to cover the same area by an 8-mm slice thickness.

Once the spiral scan is completed, the system begins to copy the acquired data into readable form so that reconstruction can begin. During this "copying phase," there is an unavoidable delay that prohibits any other function of the scanner. This delay usually lasts about 2–3 minutes.

With our particular scanner, Siemens Somatom-Plus-S, the final slice of the spiral range is reconstructed first. It is very important to see the last image in order to determine if additional scans are needed to cover any further pathology. For this reason, it is crucial that the technologist chooses to save the raw data when setting up the scan parameters. This allows the technologist to continue scanning after the spiral data have been acquired, but not reconstructed. If the raw data are not saved, extra scans cannot be taken until all the spiral images have been reconstructed. If you continued to scan before reconstructing the spiral data, all the spiral information

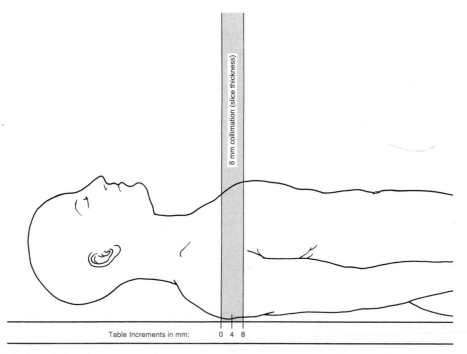

Figure 13.2. Spiral CT: 8 mm collimation scanning with 4-mm table reconstruction.

would be lost. This reconstruction time is approximately five to six images per minute. If vascular enhancement is necessary to diagnose any further pathology beyond the spiral scan, the IV contrast would have dissipated by this time. This could create the need to administer additional contrast.

The spiral data can be reconstructed at any table location. If the scan was performed using 8 mm collimation, the reconstruction interval could be set at 4 mm. This would provide overlapping images of 8 mm thick, every 4 mm.

The slice thickness cannot be changed from the original acquired thickness but the spiral data can be reconstructed at smaller table increments without additional scan time or radiation (Fig. 13.2).

Comparison

Advantages	Disadvantages
(1) Elimination of respiratory motion	(1) Low milliampere settings result in lower quality images
(2) Quick scan times (seconds)	(2) Inherent delay after spiral scan
(3) Optimal vessel opacification	(3) Maximum scan time of 40 seconds
(4) Unlimited reconstruction intervals	(4) Inability to view images as they are acquired (could lead to increased infiltrations of IV contrast)
(5) High-quality three-dimensional and multiplanar images	
(6) Reduction in IV contrast	

Two of the major disadvantages, the inherent delay and the limited scan times, will eventually be eliminated by the release and approval of the back-to-back spiral package.

Spiral CT can be used to cover any area of interest. It has become a valuable asset in the detection of abnormalities in the lungs, liver, and pancreas. Spiral scanning has provided us with information that we never believed possible in a matter of seconds. And even though there are advantages and disadvantages to spiral scanning, an important factor to remember is that not every patient is a candidate for spiral CT. The patients should be assessed for their size, breathholding ability, and the area of interest to be covered. Therefore, all these factors play an important role in determining whether or not spiral CT should be the scan method of choice (Figs. 13.3–13.11).

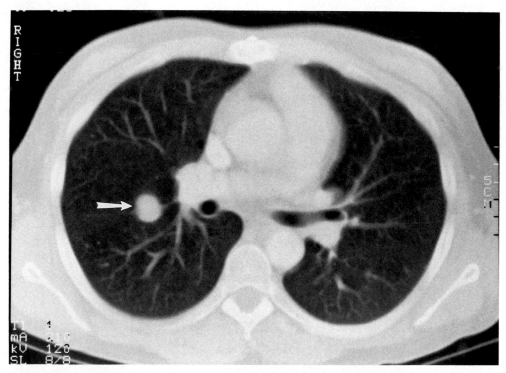

Figure 13.3. Cross-section taken at the level of the right pulmonary artery that is imaged at a lung window and level demonstrates a right lung nodule *(arrow)*. Image was acquired using a 8-mm slice and table speed and reconstructed at 4 mm table increments.

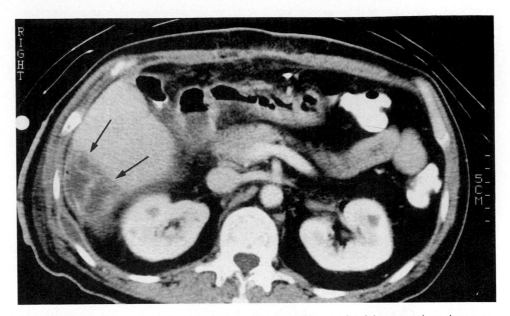

Figure 13.4. Scan acquired using an 8-mm slice and table speed and reconstructed at 8-mm table reconstruction shows multiple segmented hypodense areas *(arrows)* in the inferior position of the right lobe of the liver. This is consistent with a liver abscess.

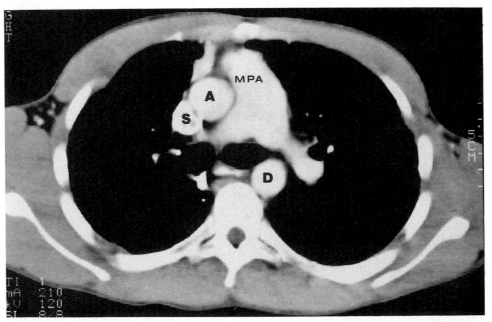

Figure 13.5. Normal cross-section of the chest exemplifies the excellent vascular opacification that can be obtained with spiral CT. *A*, aorta; *D*, descending aorta; *MPA*, main pulmonary artery; *S*, superior vena cava.

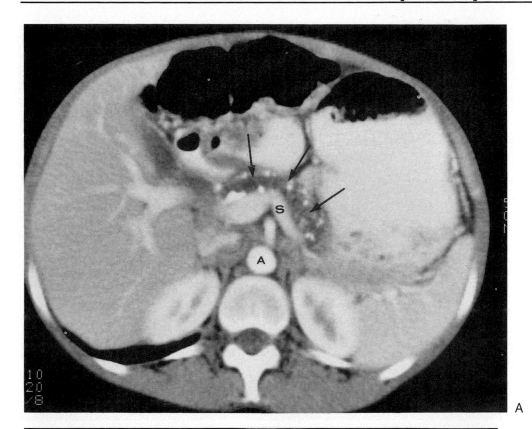

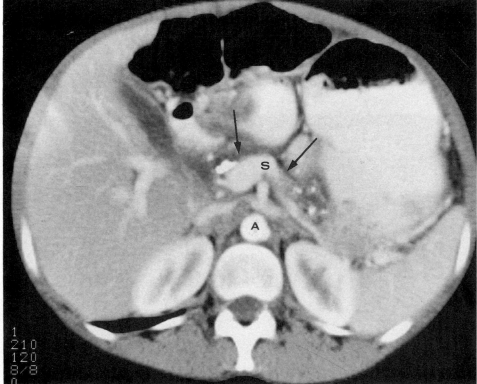

Figure 13.6. A and **B:** Consecutive images through the pancreas demonstrate a dilated pancreatic duct *(arrows)*. There is excellent vascular opacification of the aorta *(A)* and splenic vein *(S)*, which is coursing posterior to the pancreas. Images were acquired at 8-mm slice and table speed and reconstructed at table increment of 4 mm.

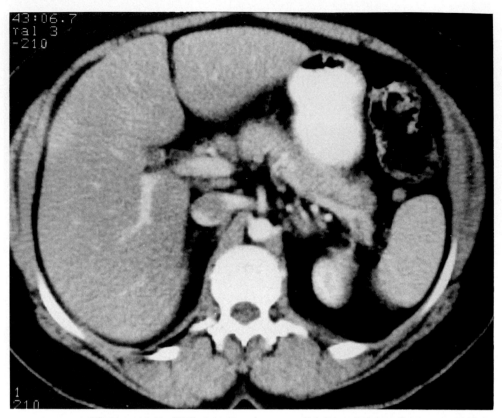

Figure 13.7. This image shows mild hepatomegaly.

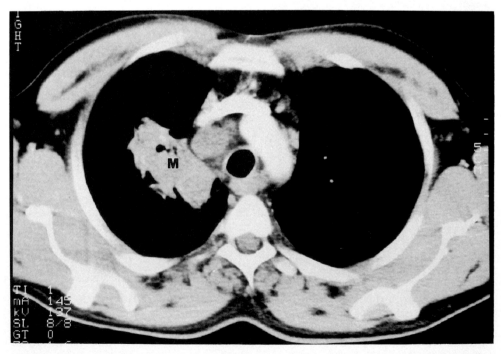

Figure 13.8. A mass *(M)* is visualized in the right upper lobe in a patient with Hodgkins' disease.

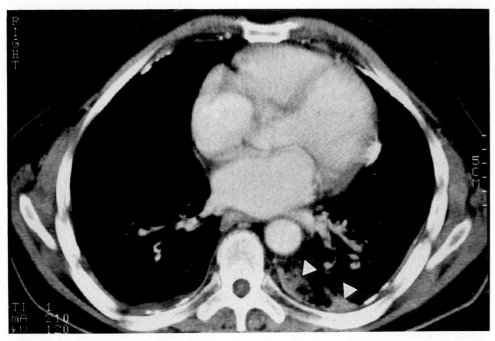

Figure 13.9. Left lower lobe *(LLL)* consolidation *(arrowheads)* is demonstrated on this image, which was acquired using a 10-mm slice, table speed, and table increment. LLL consolidation is common with pneumonia.

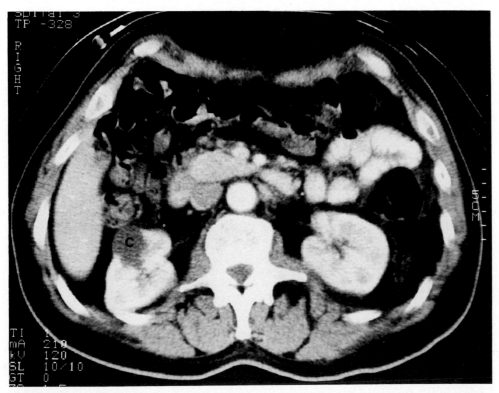

Figure 13.10. Right renal cyst. Scan through the kidneys shows a well-circumscribed, hypodense area *(C)* in the right kidney.

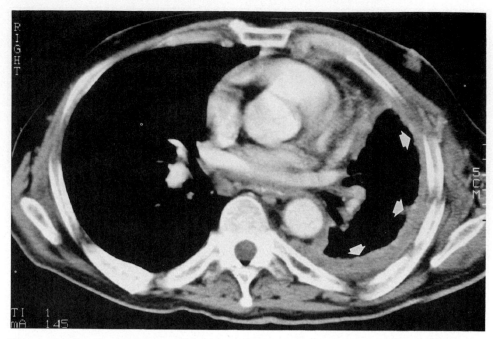

Figure 13.11. Cross-section at the level of the left atrium shows an extensive pleural process *(arrowheads)* enveloping the entire left hemithorax.

References and Suggested Readings

1. Berland L. *Practical CT: technology and techniques*. New York: Raven Press, 1987.
2. Bluemke D. *Spiral CT of the liver*. Baltimore, MD: Department of Radiology, The Johns Hopkins Institutions. 1992.
3. Fishman E, Wyatt S, Ney D, et al. *Spiral CT of the pancreas with multiplanar display*. Pictorial Essay. *Am J Roentgenol* 1992;159:1209–1215.
4. Siemens Medical Systems. Somatom Plus/Plus-S: Image Quality Guide PL C I-0I5. Issue: 04.92.

CT-Guided Interventional Techniques and General Considerations

The value of CT for performing percutaneous biopsies and abscess drainage is often overlooked. Because CT provides cross-sectional images, pathological processes are easily localized and precise catheter or needle placement can be accomplished as accurate measurements are possible, owing to the ability to see depth from the images. Use of CT for these procedures also reduces patient cost by eliminating operating expenses and additional in-patient days that might have resulted from surgery. In certain instances the examination can even be done on an out-patient basis. The risk of infection is also reduced by using CT in these examinations.

Guidelines for Percutaneous Biopsies and Fluid Aspiration/Drainage

1. A signed patient permission form is required.
2. Clotting studies should be on the chart (prothrombin time [PT]; platelet count of not more than 50% above normal). Normal PT 11–13 sec; PTT 0–35 sec.
3. A clear liquid diet is given on the day of biopsy, and the patient is given nothing by mouth (NPO) before the procedure.
4. Intravenous access is established.
5. Premedication is not routinely given except for pain control. Adequate premedication must be provided for the pediatric patient.
6. There must be surgical consultation for back-up as needed before the procedure.

187

General Technique for Percutaneous Tissue Aspiration (Cytology) or Biopsy (Histology)

1. The proper needles (Table 14.1) are chosen for cytologic aspiration or histologic biopsy. The small, 22-gauge needle is used as the first guide needle.
2. The "prep" tray (Table 14.2) is checked.

Table 14.1. *CT-guided needles for cytological and histological sampling*

1. Simple bevel needle
   a. Chiba needle (Fig. 14.3)
      Size: 23-, 22-, 20-, 18-gauge (14, 20 cm length)
      Thin-walled flexible needle with 24°–30° bevel. The 22-gauge is for cytological aspiration. The larger needle is employed for deep lesions or an obese patient.
   b. Jamshide needle
      Size 11-, 12-gauge (10 cm length)
      The cannula has a beveled tip, a flat obturator, and a very large bore for obtaining large tissue for histological analysis.
   c. Greene needle (Fig. 14.3)
      Size: 22-, 23-gauge (15 cm length) and 19-gauge (10 cm length)
      For lung biopsy. The 19-gauge needle, 10-cm needle is used first to establish a tract through the pleural membrane; then a 23-gauge thin-wall needle 15 cm long is used through the 19-gauge needle for aspiration biopsy.
   d. Meghini needle
      Size: 22-, 20-, 16-gauge (4, 6 inches length)
      The needle has a pencil-point stylet with a 45°–50° beveled cannula. The syringe has a camloc locking device for suction.
   e. Spinal needle
      Size: 22-gauge (1.5, 3, 3.5, 5, 7 inches length) and 20-gauge (1.25, 1.5, 3, 3.5 inches length.)
   f. Turner needle (Fig. 14.3)
      Size: 22-, 20-, 18-, 16-gauge (15, 20 cm length)
      The needle has a 45° bevel; the cannula is circumferentially sharpened. It cuts a core of tissue that remains inside when needle is removed.
2. Bevel needle with teeth.
   a. Franseen needle (Fig. 14.3)
      Size: 22-, 20-, 18-, 16-gauge (15, 20 cm length)
      The needle has three sharp cutting teeth that grasp the tissue when the needle is rotated.
3. Screw needle
   a. Rolex screw needle
      Size: 20-gauge (16 cm length)
      The needle contains two parts: an inner tapered screw needle and a larger outer cannula.
   b. Surgimed screw needle
      Size: 20-gauge (15 cm length)
      The instrument consists of a 23-gauge, 20-cm screw needle and a 20-gauge, 15-cm cannula.
4. Small-gauge true-cut needle
   a. Lee Trucut needle
      Size: 16.5-gauge (3, 5, 7 inch length)
   b. Westcott Trucut needle (Fig. 14.3)
      Size: 22-, 20-gauge (3.5, 5.5, 7 inch length)
      Needle is a two-piece, thin-wall needle modified to include a slotted opening.

Table 14.2. *Supplies needed for biopsy and drainage tray*

Sterile 4 × 4 inch gauze pads
Sterile poly-lined towels
Steri-drapes with aperture
Steri-strips
Sterile hemostats
Sterile scissors
Sterile gloves: size 6½, 7, 7½, 8
No. 11 scalpel blades
Syringes: 6, 10, 30, 60 cc
Needles: 18-gauge, 1.5-inch; 22-gauge, 1.5-inch; 25-gauge, 1-inch
10 Polyvinylpyrrolidone (PVP) iodine aqueous solution
Alcohol (bottle, "prep" pads)
1% Lidocaine without heparin
Saline nonbacteriostatic 30-cc vials
Extension tubing
Ruler
Surgical suture: 3-0 silk, 4-0 plain, 0-0 chromic, 0-0 silk, 4-0 silk
Bandaids

3. The patient is advised to breathe consistently and quietly during the localization and procedure. In order to avoid bending the needle and anatomical fluctuation, the patient should not breathe in and out during scanning.
4. Previous diagnostic scans are reviewed to choose the entry site. Patient position of supine or prone depends on the easiest access to the lesion. The approach with the shortest distance and requiring the least angulation is chosen.
5. Sequential scans are taken through the lesions, and the entry point is selected. The middle or solid portion of the lesion should be chosen as the entry point. Use two small opaque catheters placed over patient skin for landmarks.
6. The access site is prepared and draped. Local anesthetic is administered. The needle used for the anesthetic is left in place as a localizing marker. Depth and angulation are calculated between marker and lesion.
7. Again with quiet respiration, a 22-gauge needle is inserted into the lesion. The needle tip is then documented with CT. The tip is identified by a dark linear shadow from the needle tip. A lateral scout scan may want to be used to localize the needle tip.
8. Two-needle localization techniques are used (Fig. 14.1). Leaving the initial needle (usually 22-gauge) in place as a guide, a second needle is inserted (22-gauge or larger) adjacent to the initial needle with matching or slight angulation, especially for small lesions. Advantages of this technique are that: (1) a needle is always in place for use as a guide when making additional passes to collect more samples; (2) it is less time-consuming and more convenient; and (3) it provides tissue samples from various locations of the lesion.
9. When making the aspiration, three actions are taken at the same time: (1) advancing the needle in and out within the lesion; (2) a rotating motion clockwise and counterclockwise; and (3) simultaneous suction on the syringe (Fig. 14.2).

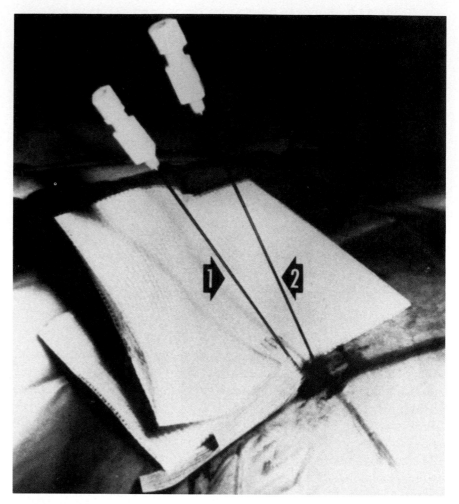

Figure 14.1. (Figs. 14.1 through 14.12 are illustrative examples of biopsy and drainage techniques that are used in various clinical situations.) Two-needle localization. The initial 22-gauge needle *(arrow 1)* is used as a guide. Note that the second needle *(arrow 2)* was inserted adjacent to the same area with slight angulation.

10. Each sample is checked for adequacy. Preferably both wet and dry samples should be obtained. A few cubic centimeters of sodium heparin are used in the needle for wet samples. Sodium heparin prevents coagulation of blood in the syringe. Water or bacteriostatic solutions, which cause lysis of the cells and inhibit bacterial growth, are avoided. A cytologist with a microscope at the site is helpful.
11. If lymphoma or multiple myeloma is suspected, a dry core sample should be obtained with a large needle (18-gauge or larger) or true cut needle (Westcott or Lee's biopsy needle).
12. Postprocedural orders are written on the chart. These should include frequent vital signs for about 1–2 hours and should be individualized as needed.
13. After a lung biopsy, scan two or more images over the region of the biopsy to evaluate for possibility of pneumothorax. Route chest x-ray on expiration 4–6 hours after lung biopsy.
14. If fluid is aspirated, appropriate studies are done (e.g., culture, Gram stain).

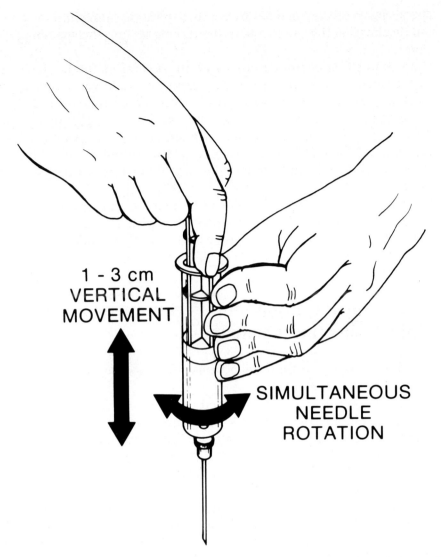

Figure 14.2. The three actions used for tissue aspiration: needle rotation, vertical movement, and suction.

Protocol for Abdominal Aspirations for Cytologic and Histologic Studies

1. Prepare an aspiration tray containing the following:
   a. Open box of albuminized slides from the refrigerator.
   b. Plastic specimen cups and lids containing 30 cc of saline.
   c. Two screw-topped coplin jars with 95% ethyl alcohol (ETOH).
   d. One screw-topped coplin jar with Carnoy's solution.
2. After tissue material has been aspirated from the patient, the needle is directed and the specimen slowly deposited onto the albuminized slide. The slide is then placed in 95% ETOH immediately.
3. If the specimen is bloody, half of the slides are immersed in Carnoy's solution until the visible blood has been lyzed. Smears should not remain in Carnoy's any longer than 5 min.

4. The syringes are cleaned out by gently aspirating saline into the needle and discharging the saline and tissue fragments into the specimen container.

5. The saline solution can be processed by several methods, depending on the specimen. Large tissue fragments are removed from the cell block preparation and the cassettes placed in formalin. If there are no tissue fragments found, the saline solution is centrifuged for 10 min at 1,500 rpm. After the initial spin, the supernatant is poured off and saved, and 95% ETOH is then added to harden the button. This tube is centrifuged again and submitted as a cell block to histologic examination.

6. The supernatant saline solution can be used for an 8 millipore filter. Smears and filters are stained with the Papanicolaou technique and mounted with Permount. The processed cell block, slides, filters, and requisition form are then given to the cytotechnologist.

General Considerations for Percutaneous Abscess or Fluid Collection Drainage

1. "Sterile" abdominal fluid collections must not be contaminated by passing through the colon.
2. If drainage is considered, CT is used to determine a safe access route so as to avoid all bowel, organs, and diaphragm.
3. Proper needles and a drainage catheter are selected before percutaneous abscess drainage (Tables 14.2 through 14.4).
4. The fluid collection and skin access are localized as for the tissue aspiration technique.
5. The fluid collection is entered using a 20-gauge needle and then aspirated. If no fluid is obtained, a larger needle is used to document its position. (An actual drainage catheter may be necessary to obtain thick pus in obvious abscesses.)
6. After initial aspiration of a few cubic centimeters of pus, the syringe is capped and sent to the laboratory for culture and Gram stain. (The area should not be aspirated completely if a drainage tube is consid-

Table 14.3. *Supplies needed for percutaneous abscess or fluid drainage*

A. Needles (Table 13.1)
  1. Chiba needle
  2. Turner needle
  3. Spinal needle, etc.
B. Guidewire (length = 88, 100, 125 cm)
  1. 0.035-inch 3 mm "J" wire
  2. 0.035-inch 15 mm "J" wire
  3. 0.038-inch 3 mm "J" wire
  4. 0.038-inch 15 mm "J" wire
C. Facial dilators: 6, 8, 10, 12 or 14F
D. Catheters (Table 13.3)
  1. Pigtail: 5, 6, 7, 8F (65, 80, 100 cm length)
  2. Polyethylene/Teflon straight or curve tip: 5–9F (50–100 cm length)
  3. Nasogastric tube: 5, 8, 10, 12, 16F (15 inches length)
E. See Table 13.2 for routine supplies

ered, as this would collapse the cavity.) At this point, the cavity is entered with a suitable guidewire through the needle. The guidewire is followed by the desired catheter, or a trocar sump drainage set (Table 14.4) is directly inserted.

7. After the catheter is placed it is secured with a tape and/or suture. The cavity is aspirated until dry and flushed with normal saline until clear.

8. Contrast and air are injected into the cavity. The cavity size and catheter location are documented with an abdominal flat plate or CT.

9. Postprocedural orders should include: (1) vital signs; and (2) catheter care (flushing of the abscess every 4–6 hours with normal saline).

10. After the drainage has lessened (4–7 days), the catheter is slowly withdrawn or replaced with a smaller catheter under fluoroscopic monitoring. The referring physician is notified regarding follow-up of the patient's condition.

Table 14.4. *Percutaneous abscess and fluid drainage kits[a]*

A. Small, medium percutaneous abscess and fluid drainage
  1. One-stick introducer system (Medi-Tech)
    a. Chiba needle with stylet (21-gauge)
    b. Cannula (6F)
    c. 0.18-inch guidewire with floppy tip
    d. 0.38-inch 3 mm "J" guidewire (100 cm)
    e. *Note:* requires self-preparation for catheter
  2. Sack one-step fluid-drain kit (Elecath)
    a. Trocar stylet†
    b. Blunt cannula (16, 18, 19 g)
    c. Pigtail catheter (5.5, 7.0, 8.2, 9.4, 11.5)[b]
    d. Retention flange
  3. Drainage catheter set for direct puncture
    a. Trocar stylet†
    b. Cannula (fit 0.038-inch guidewire)
    c. Pigtail catheter (8.3F, 25 cm length)
B. Deep and large percutaneous abscess fluid drainage
  1. Ring-McLean sump drainage set (Cook)
    a. Trocar stylet and cannula
    b. Sump catheter (12 or 16F, 30 cm length)
    c. 0.038-inch guidewire
    d. Extension tube and three-way stopcock
    e. *Note:* Requires 16-gauge introducing needle
  2. Van Sonenberg sump kit (Medi-Tech)[c]
    a. Trocar stylet and cannula
    b. Sump catheter
    c. 0.038 inch-guidewire 15 mm "J" wire (80 cm)
    d. Chiba needle (22 gauge)
    e. Sheathed needle set (18/19 gauge)
    f. Dilator
    g. Microbial air filter
    h. Suction adapter
    i. Adhesive pads
    j. Three-way stopcock

[a] These are only examples in the table; other systems are available as well.
[b] Catheter length averages 20.5 cm.
[c] Catheter: 12F (30 cm long), 14F (30 cm long).

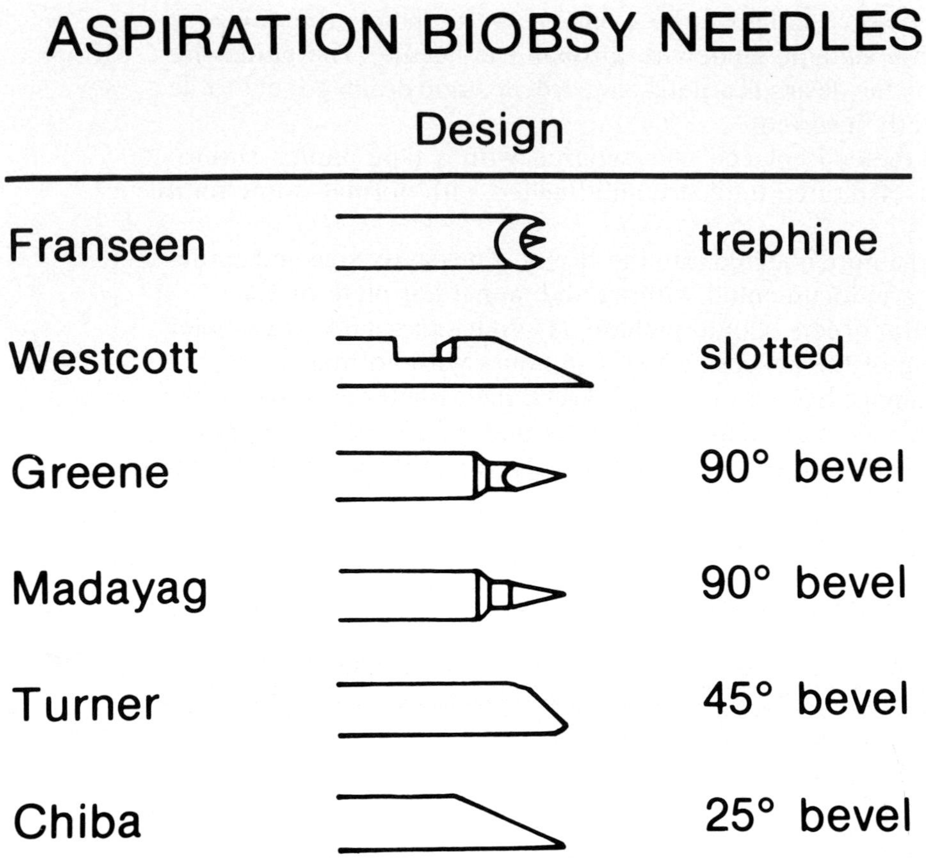

ASPIRATION BIOBSY NEEDLES

Design

Franseen		trephine
Westcott		slotted
Greene		90° bevel
Madayag		90° bevel
Turner		45° bevel
Chiba		25° bevel

Figure 14.3. Selected needles often used in CT-guided percutaneous tissue aspiration and biopsies.

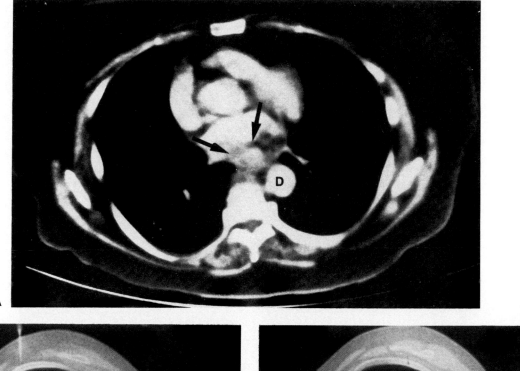

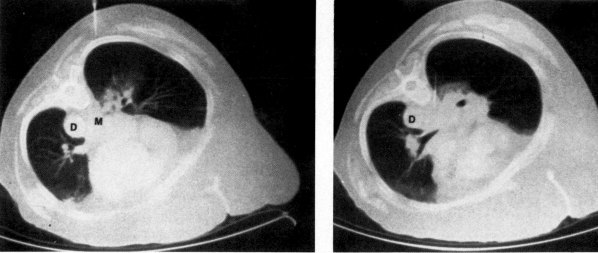

Figure 14.4. Needle-directed biopsy of the mediastinum in a patient with bladder carcinoma. **(A)** Mediastinal mass *(arrows)* anterior to the vertebral body. *D,* descending aorta. **(B)** The patient is in a left decubitus position. Note that the needle is positioned so the shortest and most direct route to the lesion *(M)* is used. **(C)** The tip of the needle has been accurately placed into the mass, which is between the descending aorta and the right pulmonary artery. Biopsy of the mass revealed metastatic disease.

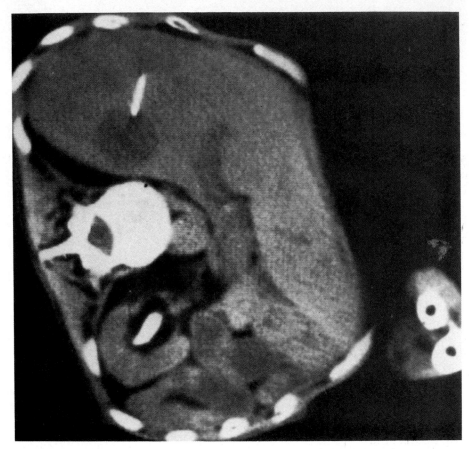

Figure 14.5. Biopsy using the posterior transthoracic approach. This patient was unable to lie in the prone position because of obstructive lung disease. Tissue samples from the mass revealed lung carcinoma.

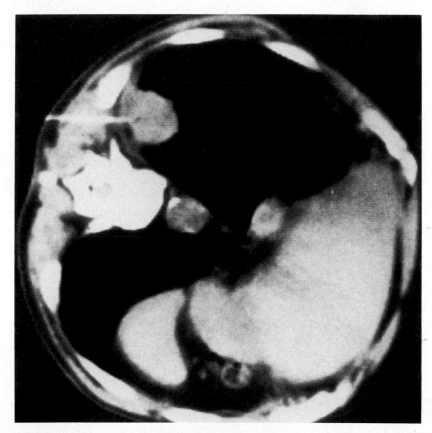

Figure 14.6. Liver tissue aspiration. In this case, the entry was chosen from the right side of the abdomen with the patient in a left decubitus position. This approach was chosen because of the shorter distance. A posterior approach was not used because of the presence of lung and diaphragm. This lesion turned out to be an abscess.

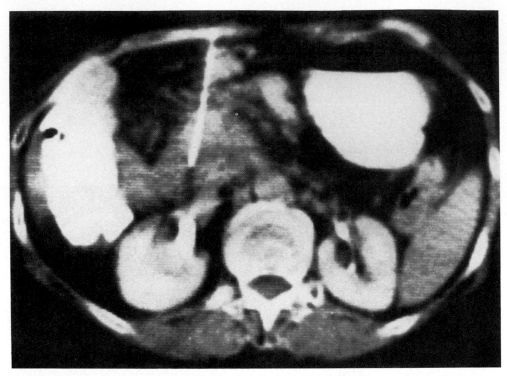

Figure 14.7. Direct anterior abdominal approach. Note the typical shadowing from the tip of the needle within the head of the pancreas. Laboratory results proved this mass to be pancreatic carcinoma.

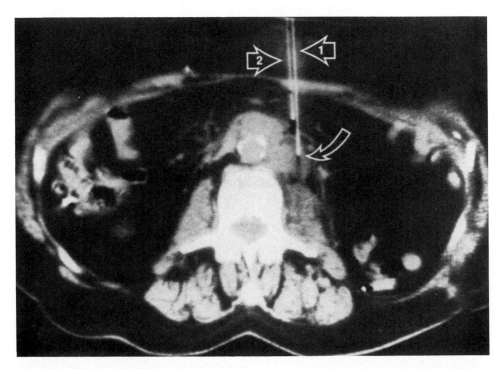

Figure 14.8. Two-needle technique. The tip of needle 1 *(curved arrow)* is seen within the lesion. Needle 2 is inserted parallel and medial to needle 1, which is being used as a guide. This mass represented metastatic nodes from transitional cell carcinoma of the bladder.

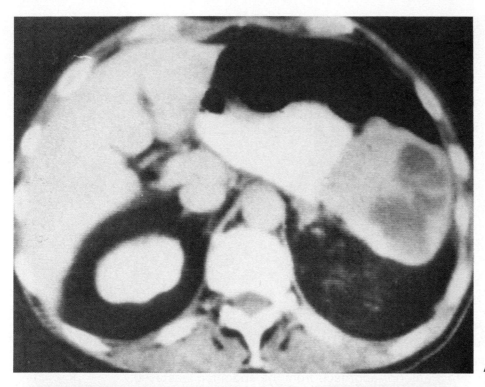

A

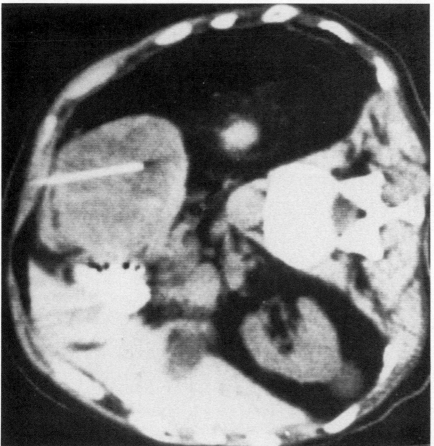

B

Figure 14.9. Islet cell carcinoma of the pancreas. **(A)** Note the dilated colon ventral and lateral to a large pancreatic tail mass. **(B)** Right decubitus scan shows that the colon has shifted to the left side, making a direct anterior approach possible.

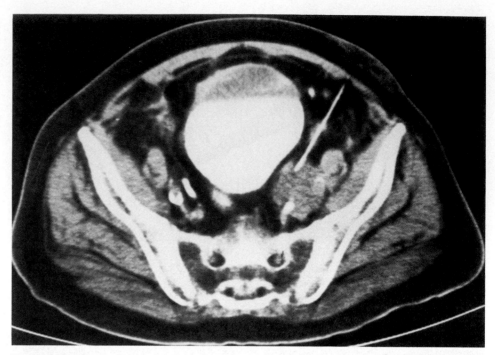

Figure 14.10. Left inguinal nodes from a patient with carcinoma of the cervix. A direct anterior approach from the abdomen was used.

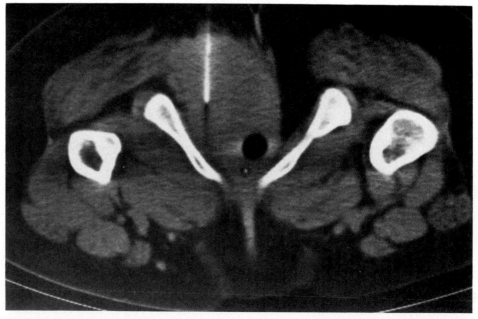

Figure 14.11. Rhadomyosarcoma of the vagina. This approach was made from the posterior buttock with the patient in the prone position.

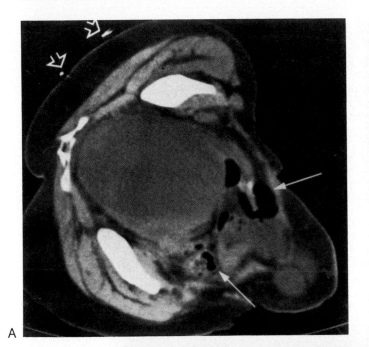

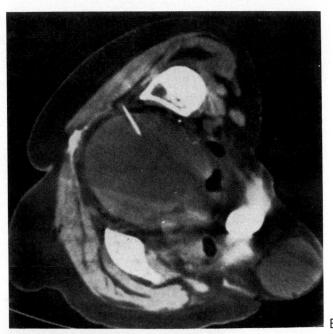

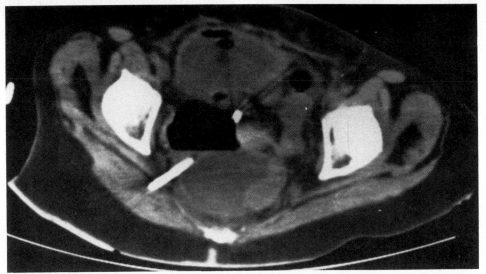

Figure 14.12. Pelvic abscess drainage. **(A)** The abscess was drained with the patient in a left decubitus position and using a right posterior buttock approach because of distended bowel *(long arrow)* and extreme obesity. Note the needle markers *(open arrows)* on the skin surface. **(B)** An 18-gauge needle was inserted into the large abscess cavity. **(C)** Subsequently a drainage catheter was placed, and 800 cc of pus was removed. There has been a marked reduction in the size of the abscess, which is outlined by air, which was injected through the catheter.

References and Suggested Readings

1. Barth KH, Matsumoto AH. Patient care in interventional radiology: a perspective. *Radiology* 1991;178:11–17.
2. Charboneau JW, Reading CC, Welch TJ. CT and sonographically guided needle biopsy: current techniques and new innovations. *Am J Roetgenol* 1990;154:1–10.
3. Ferrucci JT, Wittenberg J, Mueller PR, et al. Diagnosis of abdominal malignancy by radiologic fine-needle aspiration biopsy. *Am J Roetgenol* 1980;134:323–330.
4. Gazelle GS, Haaga JR. Guided percutaneous biopsy of intraabdominal lesions. *Am J Roetgenol* 1989;153:929–935.
5. Gazelle GS, Haaga JR, Stellato TA, et al. *Pelvic abscesses: CT-guided transrectal drainage. Radiology* 1991;181:49–51.
6. Haaga JR. New techniques for CT-guided biopsies. *Am J Roetgenol* 1979;133:633–641.
7. Kane NM, Korobkin M, Francis IR, et al. Percutaneous biopsy of left adrenal masses: prevalence of pancreatitis after anterior approach. *Am J Roetgenol* 1991;157:777–780.
8. Palestrant AM. Comprehensive approach to CT-guided procedures with a hand-held guidance device. *Radiology* 1990;174:270–272.
9. Smith EH. Complication of percutaneous abdominal fine-needle biopsy. *Radiology* 1991;178:253–258.

Subject Index

Subject Index